Multiple Choice Questions in Haematology

T P Baglin, PhD MRCP MRCPath
Haematologist, Addenbrooke's Hospital, Cambridge

J E G Braithwaite, MA MRCP MRCPath
Haematologist, James Paget Hospital, Great Yarmouth

T R Mitchell, MA MD FRCPath
Haematologist, James Paget Hospital, Great Yarmouth

Edward Arnold
A division of Hodder & Stoughton
LONDON   MELBOURNE   AUCKLAND

Contents

	Question	Page
General haematology	1–5	2–5
Hypochromic and normochromic anaemias	6–19	6–13
Macrocytic anaemia	20–31	14–20
Haemolytic anaemia	32–49	20–32
White cells and HIV infection	50–62	32–41
Leukaemias	63–80	42–54
Multiple myeloma	81–84	55–58
Lymphomas	85–89	58–61
Aplastic anaemia and pancytopenia	90–92	62–63
Myeloproliferative and myelodysplastic disorders	93–98	64–68
The spleen	99–101	68–70
Coagulation and bleeding disorders	102–130	70–95
Blood transfusion and blood products	131–140	96–109

Preface

The objective of this book is to assist the revision and learning of haematology. This subject is rapidly expanding with constantly changing concepts. We have therefore kept the answers completely up-to-date, so that the content of some of the explanations may not, as yet, have appeared in the current text books.

After careful validation we feel the book will be useful to undergraduates and postgraduates, especially trainees facing the MRCP, MRCPath or other higher qualifying examinations. It should also be of value to those taking the IMLS examinations.

How to use this book

The main topics are set out in the Contents page. Every question consists of a stem and five statements, which must be judged true or false. It is suggested that all the questions on a given page are considered before reading the opposite page, where the answers and explanations are set out. The questions may be tackled by an individual but multiple choice questions do lend themselves to small group learning and revision.

Acknowledgements

We would like to thank all those who have helped with validation. Thanks also to Elizabeth Cousson who typed and collated the final draft together with Kim Llewellyn and Ashling McColgan who deciphered the original handwritten draft into a usable form.

Dedication

We would like to dedicate this book both to our families and the late Professor Geoffrey Pegrum, who was co-author of the first edition.

1   The following are statements concerning genetic factors related to haematology:
    (a) Half the children of parents who both have sickle trait will be anaemic.
    (b) The Xga blood group is inherited as a sex-linked character. All the sons of an
         Xg(a+) father and Xg(a−) mother will be Xg(a+).
    (c) Neutrophil 'drumsticks' are usually found in Turner syndrome.
    (d) A Rhesus-negative gravida 3 mother (Rhesus genotype cde/cde) has
         had one stillborn child due to Rhesus (anti-D) haemolytic disease. Her
         husband's probable genotype is CDe/cde. The risk of having an affected
         child in the next pregnancy is one in four.
    (e) Some Down's Sydrome sufferers have 46 chromosomes.

2   Which of the following statements concerning haemopoiesis are correct?
    (a) Pluripotent haemopoietic stem cells (PHSC) can be grown in semisolid agar
         cultures.
    (b) Pluripotent haemopoietic stem cells are sensitive to modulation by
         granulocyte/macrophage colony stimulating factor (GM-CSF).
    (c) The pronormoblast is a target cell for erythropoietin (Epo).
    (d) The bone marrow stromal cells have no defined role.
    (e) The lymphocyte progenitor cell arises independently of the PHSC.

1 (a) **False**   Each parent has one β^s gene and one normal β gene. Therefore the probability is that only one child in four will inherit the β^s gene from both parents ($\beta^s\beta^s$). There is a one in two chance of a child having sickle cell trait and a one in four chance of not inheriting any β^s gene ($\beta\beta$).

   (b) **False**   All the sons will be Xg(a−) as they will inherit their X chromosome from their mother.

   (c) **False**   The presence of a 'drumstick' indicates that two X chromosomes are present. In Turner's syndrome (XO) drumsticks are absent.

   (d) **False**   Each parent will pass on half of their Rhesus genotype intact because the gene complex is closely associated on chromosome 1. The chance of a child inheriting the D antigen is therefore one in two.

   (e) **True**   Although the most common form is due to non-dysjunction of chromosome 21 yielding 47 chromosomes, 3–5% of cases have a translocation of chromosome 21 to chromosome 14. This can be demonstrated by chromosome 'banding' techniques. Down's syndrome is associated with a ten-fold increase in the likelihood of acute leukaemia.

2 (a) **False**   The mouse spleen colony assay is the only reliable means of growing colonies from PHSC. If the haemopoietic tissue of a mouse is destroyed by irradiation, subsequent injection of marrow cells from a syngeneic mouse results in visible colonies forming in the irradiated mouse's spleen. The colonies comprise all the elements of haemopoiesis. PHSC in humans are only presumed to exist.

   (b) **False**   The factors controlling pluripotent stem cell renewal and differentiation are as yet ill-defined. Multi-CSF (previously recognised as interleukin 3) stimulates progenitor cells that give rise to all the elements of haemopoiesis.

   (c) **True**   Epo accelerates division of erythroblasts at all stages. High levels of Epo shorten erythroid precursor cell cycle and marrow transit times. However, the prime target of Epo is the cell membrane of the committed erythroid stem cell (CFU-E) which is triggered into cell cycle and by division gives rise to pronormoblasts. This presumably necessitates a secondary response by the PHSC to replenish the CFU-E compartment.

   (d) **False**   The stromal cells of the marrow constitute the 'microenvironment' and whilst collectively they clearly support haemopoiesis, the precise contribution of the different components is not known. One function is thought to be the presentation of cytokines to the various stem cells of the haemopoietic superstructure.

   (e) **False**   There is compelling evidence that the lymphoid progenitor cell, as well as the myeloid progenitor cell, is a derivative of the PHSC.

3 Which of the following statements relating to erythropoietin (Epo) are correct?
   (a) It is usually decreased in patients with high affinity haemoglobins.
   (b) It is increased in patients with congenital 2,3-diphosphoglycerate (2,3-DPG) deficiency.
   (c) Oestrogen facilitates the production of erythropoietin.
   (d) Plasma levels are often reduced in chronic renal failure.
   (e) Therapeutic venesection may be required after a renal transplant.

4 The following compensatory mechanisms occur in severe anaemia (i.e. haemoglobin concentration < 6 g/dl):
   (a) Arterial Pao_2 is decreased.
   (b) Red cell 2,3-diphosphoglycerate (2,3-DPG) increases.
   (c) There is an increase in cardiac output at rest.
   (d) The concentration of erythropoietin in the urine is often increased.
   (e) Whole blood viscosity is increased.

5 The following relate to the symptoms of severe chronic anaemia:
   (a) Skin pallor can be absent.
   (b) Swelling of the ankles can occur.
   (c) The peripheral pulses can be 'collapsing' in type.
   (d) Shortness of breath on exertion is rare.
   (e) Angina pectoris can be troublesome.

3 (a) **False** The oxygen dissociation curve is shifted to the left, thus limiting oxygen delivery to the tissues. This relative hypoxia will stimulate erythropoietin production by the kidneys.

   (b) **True** 2,3-DPG is the major regulator of oxygen affinity and reduces the high affinity of haemoglobin for oxygen by several mechanisms. Thus 2,3-DPG deficiency reduces oxygen delivery to the tissues, stimulating Epo production.

   (c) **False** Oestrogen reduces Epo production and also antagonises its effect. This may be a factor in the differential between mean haemoglobin concentration in men and women.

   (d) **True** Due to the destruction of normal renal tissue.

   (e) **True** Erythropoietin production is sometimes inappropriately increased after renal allografting. Occasionally the haemoglobin increases sufficiently to warrant venesection. The mechanism for this is unclear but the patient's own diseased kidneys may be the source of Epo production as removal of the native kidneys corrects the polycythaemia.

4 (a) **False** Unless there is a pre-existing perfusion/diffusion defect in the lungs, Pao_2 is maintained within the normal range.

   (b) **True** In most anaemias 2,3-DPG concentration is increased. This causes a shift to the right of the oxygen dissociation curve and facilitates oxygen delivery to the tissues.

   (c) **True** This is a later event in anaemia. The haemoglobin concentration usually falls below 6–7 g/dl before cardiac output is consistently increased at rest.

   (d) **True** In most anaemias the reduction in oxygen tension in the renal tissues causes increased production of renal erythropoietin with elevated levels in the plasma and urine.

   (e) **False** Whole blood viscosity is decreased and the peripheral resistance reduced.

5 (a) **True** Skin pallor is influenced by the amount of circulating haemoglobin, the degree of skin vasoconstriction and skin pigmentation. Although a reduction in skin blood flow is common, it may be modified by other factors, including the ambient temperature and hypoxia. Pallor is best detected by examination of the conjunctivae and the mucous membranes of the mouth.

   (b) **True** This may herald congestive cardiac failure but slight ankle oedema can sometimes be found in its absence.

   (c) **True** As the haemoglobin falls progressively below 6-7 g/dl, cardiac output increases. The resultant clinical features will depend upon age and the state of the cardiovascular system. In young patients without heart disease a high output state occurs with a hyperdynamic circulation characterised by a collapsing pulse and dilated peripheral vessels. In the elderly, and in those with heart disease, the myocardium cannot sustain the high output and cardiac failure ensues.

   (d) **False** Although an increased ventilatory rate serves little purpose in the absence of pulmonary disease, it is a common symptom. It is due to vagal stimulation subsequent upon the increased venous filling pressure seen in the pulmonary circulation.

   (e) **True** Particularly in the elderly and those with pre-existing heart disease.

6   The following statements relate to the gain and loss of iron in the body:
    (a) Absorption of iron takes place only in the lower part of the small intestine.
    (b) In adult males at least 4 mg of iron is lost from the body each day.
    (c) The average iron loss during each menstrual period is 120–150 mg.
    (d) Iron requirements in pregnancy are increased.
    (e) Adult males absorb about 1 mg of iron from the diet each day.

7   Which of the following statements concerning iron metabolism are correct?
    (a) Free iron is found in the circulating blood.
    (b) Serum ferritin is in equilibrium with the ferritin in the body iron stores.
    (c) The serum iron concentration is always low in iron deficiency.
    (d) Iron within the body is mainly present in the reticuloendothelial system.
    (e) More than 95% of the iron used for erythropoiesis is obtained from red cell
         breakdown.

8   The following concern the clinical features of iron deficiency anaemia:
    (a) The patient can be totally asymptomatic.
    (b) Atrophic glossitis is a very common symptom.
    (c) Iron is essential for normal nail growth.
    (d) Pica may occur.
    (e) Splenomegaly is a common clinical finding.

9   Which of the following are consistent with a diagnosis of chronic iron deficiency?
    (a) Haemoglobin 6.0 g/dl, mean corpuscular volume (MCV) 60 fl, mean corpus-
         cular haemoglobin (MCH) 18.5 pg.
    (b) A serum ferritin of 4 μg/l (normal 15–300 μg/l).
    (c) An absolute reticulocyte count of 150 × 10^9/l (30–100 × 10^9/l).
    (d) A reduced serum transferrin concentration.
    (e) A platelet count of 660 × 10^9/l.

6 (a) **False**   Iron is absorbed in the duodenum and upper jejunum.
  (b) **False**   Each day 0.2–0.3 mg of iron is lost from the skin; average gut loss is 0.4 mg as blood and 0.2 mg in epithelial cells and bile; less than 0.1 mg per day is lost in the urine: a total of 0.9–1.0 mg per day.
  (c) **False**   The average amount of blood lost during each period is 30 ml, representing 12–15 mg of iron.
  (d) **True**   Approximately 750 mg of iron is required to provide fetal and extra maternal needs.
  (e) **True**   Only 5–10% of dietary iron (10–15 mg/day in a western diet) is absorbed.

7 (a) **False**   All circulating iron is bound to transferrin. Free ionic iron is highly toxic and will give rise to iron poisoning.
  (b) **True**   Serum ferritin is the most clinically useful index of body iron stores in normal subjects and most disease states.
  (c) **False**   The first stage in developing the iron lack is a fall in iron stores (prelatent iron deficiency). Only when the stores are depleted does the serum iron concentration diminish, although the haemoglobin may still be normal at this stage (latent iron deficiency).
  (d) **False**   Iron is mainly present in the form of haemoglobin (2.5 g in a 70 kg man). Mobilisable iron stores in the reticuloendothelial tissues amount to 0.6–0.9 g in males, less in females.
  (e) **True**   The body is very efficient at conserving iron.

8 (a) **True**   The onset can be very insidious. Symptoms of tiredness and lethargy may not appear until the haemoglobin has diminished to 9–10 g/dl.
  (b) **False**   Loss of the filiform papillae occurs in less than 40% of patients, usually the elderly. Glossitis may be accompanied by angular cheilosis.
  (c) **True**   However, clinically evident nail dystrophy (e.g. ridging, koilonychia) resulting from iron deficiency is seen infrequently.
  (d) **True**   The eating of earth or clay, especially in children, may aggravate or even cause deficiency due to adsorption of food iron, rendering it unavailable for absorption. Other forms of pica are common, e.g. pagophagia (ice eating) in adults.
  (e) **False**   Slight splenomegaly may be found in children with iron deficiency, but if it occurs in adults other causes should be sought.

9 (a) **True**   This is a hypochromic, microcytic blood picture typical of iron deficiency.
  (b) **True**   Reflecting absent body iron stores.
  (c) **False**   Due to the absence of iron stores a reticulocyte response is absent. It may be found once treatment has commenced.
  (d) **False**   Serum transferrin is raised in iron deficiency.
  (e) **True**   Thrombocytosis is a common response to bleeding but may also be seen in some patients without evidence of blood loss.

10 A 40-year-old woman presents with a hypochromic microcytic anaemia that fails to respond to treatment with oral iron. Which of the following should be considered as possible causes?
  (a) Poor diet.
  (b) A previous partial gastrectomy.
  (c) Gluten-induced enteropathy.
  (d) That the anaemia has been wrongly diagnosed.
  (e) An underlying carcinoma of the colon.

11 A 43-year-old asthmatic with menorrhagia is admitted from the waiting list for hysterectomy. Her haemoglobin is found to be 8.2 g/dl. The anaesthetist refuses to consider her for operation on the grounds that her haemoglobin is < 10 g/dl. Which of the following statements are correct?
  (a) Her operation should proceed following a blood transfusion.
  (b) Intravenous total dose infusion of iron is contraindicated.
  (c) Her haemoglobin is likely to increase by 6 g/dl over the subsequent 3 weeks if she is given oral iron therapy.
  (d) Iron therapy should be continued for 3 months after the operation.
  (e) A progestogen preparation may be useful.

12 The following are causes of a suboptimal or slow response to iron treatment:
  (a) Some iron preparations.
  (b) Non-compliance.
  (c) Dermatitis herpetiformis.
  (d) Coexisting infection.
  (e) Hyperthyroidism.

10 (a) **False**   Dietary iron would be a minor factor during the administration of oral iron.

   (b) **True**   Iron absorption is impaired by lack of acid secretion and perhaps increased bowel transit time.

   (c) **True**   Malabsorption should always be considered when a patient fails to respond to iron.

   (d) **True**   There are other causes of hypochromic microcytic anaemia.

   (e) **True**   Even if there are no symptoms, occult blood studies should always be performed in this age group. Even if these are negative, if no other cause of the iron deficiency can be found then further investigation of the gastrointestinal tract is essential.

11 (a) **False**   Blood transfusion is potentially hazardous when compared with alternative treatment strategies.

   (b) **True**   This should never be given where there is a history of allergy.

   (c) **False**   The optimal rate of rise of haemoglobin on oral iron is 0.15–0.25 g/dl per day (approximately 1 g/week). The patient has menorrhagia, which is likely to limit the response.

   (d) **True**   The objective is to increase the haemoglobin concentration to normal and replace the patient's reticuloendothelial iron stores.

   (e) **True**   A preparation such as norethisterone may arrest menstrual bleeding in the short-term and, together with oral iron therapy, will allow the haemoglobin concentration to rise to levels compatible with anaesthesia/surgery.

12 (a) **True**   In some individuals with faster than average bowel transit times, slow release iron preparations fail to present iron to the duodenum and upper jejunum.

   (b) **True**   Common and often due to gastrointestinal intolerance. Compliance can be assessed by enquiry as to the stool colour and in most circumstances by a random serum iron measurement.

   (c) **True**   This skin condition is associated with gluten-induced enteropathy.

   (d) **True**   Iron delivery to the erythroid precursors is reduced in the presence of infection or inflammation.

   (e) **False**   The response to iron deficiency is not affected by thyroid overactivity. Conversely, incomplete responses can be seen in patients with hypothyroidism unless they receive simultaneous thyroxine therapy.

13 A fit 38-year-old woman of English ancestry is found on a routine screen to have the following blood results: haemoglobin 12.1 g/dl, white cell count 6.8 × 10⁹/l, platelets 183 × 10⁹/l, MCV 65.2 fl, MCH 19.6 pg, reticulocytes 30 × 10⁹/l and plasma viscosity 1.50 mPAs (at 25°C) (normal 1.5–1.72 mPAs). Her serum ferritin is 58 μg/l (normal 15–300 μg/l). Which of the following diagnoses might explain these results?
   (a) Latent iron deficiency.
   (b) Congenital sideroblastic anaemia.
   (c) Idiopathic haemochromatosis.
   (d) beta thalassaemia minor.
   (d) Haemoglobin H disease.

14 The following statements relate to ferritin:
   (a) The serum concentration may be in the normal range in iron deficient individuals receiving oral iron.
   (b) It behaves as an acute-phase protein.
   (c) The serum concentration is high in untreated haemochromatosis.
   (d) Serum concentrations are usually low in alcoholic liver disease.
   (e) Low serum concentrations are found in 4-week-old infants.

15 The following are statements relating to the erythrocyte sedimentation rate (ESR) and plasma viscosity (PV):
   (a) The ESR is high if carried out on defibrinated blood.
   (b) Chronic-phase protein reactions increase plasma viscosity.
   (c) Plasma viscosity is dependent upon the haematocrit.
   (d) The ESR is likely to be normal 24 h after the onset of lobar pneumonia.
   (e) A plasma viscosity > 2.5 mPAs at 25°C is most likely to be caused by the presence of a paraprotein.

13 (a) **False**   A normal ferritin without an acute phase response (normal viscosity) indicates that iron stores are adequate.

(b) **False**   This condition is usually inherited as a sex-linked condition presenting earlier in life.

(c) **False**   Iron overload is reflected by a raised ferritin. There is no anaemia. Iron inclusion bodies (Pappenheimer bodies) may be present in circulating red cells.

(d) **True**   A characteristic picture of a moderate hypochromic microcytic blood picture with a normal haemoglobin and iron stores. The spontaneous mutation rate of this condition in the British population is approximately 1 per 100 000.

(e) **False**   Haemolysis in this patient is unlikely with a normal reticulocyte count. In addition, the condition is usually found in Asians. Haemoglobin H disease is characterised by a mild to moderate chronic haemolytic anaemia with hypochromic microcytic red cells. It results from deletion or mutation of three of the four alpha globin (alpha thalassaemia) genes. Haemoglobin H refers to $\beta 4$ tetramers.

14 (a) **True**   Although the major part of the iron absorbed is bound to transferrin and utilised by the developing red cells, a small proportion enters the iron storage pool. A blood sample for serum ferritin taken during iron therapy will therefore not necessarily confirm the diagnosis of iron deficiency.

(b) **True**   Serum ferritin increases after trauma, operations and after transient infection.

(c) **True**   Generally reflecting the degree of iron overload, commonly 20 g or more.

(d) **False**   The ferritin concentration is often at the upper end of the normal range. It then increases in proportion to the degree of liver damage unless bleeding supervenes.

(e) **True**   At birth, cord levels correlate with maternal ferritin but as the red cells associated with the erythrocytosis of the newborn become senescent, ferritin concentration rises (mean 350 μg/l). The mean concentration falls during the next 6 months to about 30 μg/l.

15 (a) **False**   Fibrinogen is the main plasma protein factor that controls red cell rouleau formation, which in turn determines the rate of fall of red cells in the ESR tube.

(b) **True**   When the chronic phase proteins (e.g. fibrinogen and immunoglobulin) are increased, both the PV and ESR are increased.

(c) **False**   The test is carried out on the supernatant plasma of a spun sample. This independence from red cell factors gives superiority over the ESR, which is affected by the haematocrit and red cell size, shape and agglutination.

(d) **False**   The acute phase reaction proteins (fibrinogen, C-reactive protein, α_2-macroglobulin, etc.) are usually increased 24 h after the onset of infection, injury, infarction or inflammation.

(e) **True**   The presence of a paraprotein increases the PV and ESR. Any patient with an increase in PV of > 2.5 mPAs should have a protein electrophoresis performed.

16 The following statements relate to anaemias secondary to chronic disorders (ASCD):
   (a) The red cell life-span is reduced.
   (b) Serum ferritin levels are decreased.
   (c) Erythropoietin levels are high.
   (d) The MCH is characteristically reduced.
   (e) Plasma viscosity is usually increased.

17 The following haematology results were obtained from a 59-year-old female patient: haemoglobin 10 g/dl, MCV 75 fl, MCH 25 pg, white blood count 2.2 × 10⁹/l (neutrophils 0.8 × 10⁹/l), platelets 151 × 10⁹/l. Plasma viscosity 2.02 mPAs (normal 1.5–1.72 mPAs), serum ferritin 44 μg/l (normal 15-150 μg/l). These results could be found in:
   (a) Pernicious anaemia.
   (b) Felty's syndrome.
   (c) Miliary tuberculosis.
   (d) Cushing's disease.
   (e) Oat-cell carcinoma of the lung.

18 The following are statements concerning some of the haematological findings during pregnancy:
   (a) The haemoglobin concentration decreases.
   (b) The red cell mass decreases.
   (c) A white cell count of 20 × 10⁹/l following delivery is common.
   (d) The platelet count usually decreases by week 30.
   (e) The fetus takes priority over the mother in the demand for iron.

19 The following are further statements relating to the haematological changes occurring in pregnancy:
   (a) The MCV is increased.
   (b) The serum ferritin concentration falls.
   (c) Serum B_{12} is elevated.
   (d) A patient with the following results: haemoglobin 9.9 g/dl, MCV 84 fl, MCH 28 pg, cannot be iron-deficient.
   (e) Folate deficiency is common in pregnant British women.

16 (a) **True** There is a modest reduction in red cell life to 80–90 days.

 (b) **False** Ferritin concentration is normal or increased, probably due to iron stored as a consequence of (a). The serum iron is low and transferrin normal or reduced.

 (c) **False** Epo concentrations tend to be low. This may explain the failure of the marrow to respond to the anaemia but the precise mechanisms are complex and unclarified.

 (d) **True** The red cell indices (MCV/MCH) are characteristically those of a mild hypochromic microcytic anaemia but may be normal.

 (e) **True** Due to the chronic-phase protein reaction.

17 (a) **False** The blood picture should be macrocytic.

 (b) **True** Felty's syndrome comprises rheumatoid arthritis (RA), splenomegaly and neutropenia. The mild anaemia has the characteristics of ASCD and is typical of RA.

 (c) **True** ASCD would be expected in this condition. Neutropenia is a rare but well-documented complication.

 (d) **False** Cushing's disease is usually characterised by a small increase in red cell mass and a neutrophilia.

 (e) **True** Malignancies are often accompanied by ASCD. Neutropenia may be a manifestation of bone marrow infiltration.

18 (a) **True** There is a progressive fall in haemoglobin concentration of 2 g/dl. It starts at 12–16 weeks and in normal circumstances rarely falls below the concentration reached at 26–28 weeks.

 (b) **False** The red cell mass increases by 10-20% (average 250 ml) and the plasma volume by about 50% (average 1250 ml) but there is a good deal of variation between individuals and parity in the same individual. The WHO defines anaemia in pregnancy as < 10 g/dl but the variation above explains some haemoglobin concentrations around 10 g/dl without obvious cause except haemodilution.

 (c) **True** The total number of white cells is increased during pregnancy due to a greater proportion of neutrophils. The count is usually about 12–15 × 10⁹/l but at delivery, because of blood loss and trauma, it frequently rises to 20 × 10⁹/l.

 (d) **False** There is no consistent change in platelet count. However, 5–10% of pregnant women develop mild thrombocytopenia for no apparent reason other than pregnancy.

 (e) **True** The placenta has iron receptors with even greater affinity for iron than maternal transferrin.

19 (a) **True** There is a physiological increase of 4–5 fl or even more. The mechanism is obscure.

 (b) **True** The concentration falls continuously during the first 32 weeks and then plateaus at either the lower end of the normal or in the iron deficient range. This is due to the maternal red cell mass increment and fetal demand.

 (c) **False** Serum B_{12} falls progressively during pregnancy due to fetal demand and haemodilution.

 (d) **False** The normal macrocytosis of pregnancy may mask the development of iron deficiency.

 (e) **False** Both serum and red cell folate concentrations diminish during pregnancy but deficiency is rare in populations with an adequate dietary intake.

20 The following concern vitamin B_{12}:
   (a) It is plentiful in a mixed diet, so inadequate intake is rare.
   (b) The daily requirement of vitamin B_{12} is about 100 μg.
   (c) The body stores of vitamin B_{12} are present in sufficient amounts to last 2–3 years.
   (d) The most common cause of vitamin B_{12} deficiency in the UK is lack of intrinsic factor production.
   (e) Vitamin B_{12} is absorbed in the upper jejunum.

21 The following statements are about folic acid:
   (a) The folic acid content of food is unaffected by cooking.
   (b) The body stores will last for 4 months if folate intake is markedly reduced.
   (c) Folic acid is absorbed in the ileum.
   (d) Serum folate gives a good indication of the quantity of folic acid present in the body.
   (e) Folic acid requirements are increased by haemolysis.

22 The following concern the action of vitamin B_{12} and/or folic acid:
   (a) Folic acid is required for normal DNA synthesis.
   (b) The skin, nails and hair are most affected by B_{12} deficiency.
   (c) Folic acid lack is associated with peripheral neuropathy.
   (d) Vitamin B_{12} deficiency produces patchy demyelination in peripheral nerves.
   (e) The brain is not involved in B_{12} deficiency.

23 A 55-year-old previously fit male presents to his GP with lack of energy. A full blood count reveals a haemoglobin of 13.8 g/dl, MCV 106 fl, WBC 8.8 x 10^9/l and platelets 181 x 10^9/l. Which of the following diagnoses should be considered?
   (a) Excessive alcohol intake.
   (b) Gastrointestinal bleeding.
   (c) Hypothyroidism.
   (d) Carcinoma of the prostate.
   (e) Aplastic anaemia.

24 Red cell macrocytosis occurs regularly during treatment with the following drugs:
   (a) Hydroxyurea.
   (b) Azidothymidine (AZT).
   (c) Oral contraceptives.
   (d) Methotrexate.
   (e) Chlorothiazide diuretics.

20 (a) **True**   Only strict vegans are at risk of having a deficient diet.
   (b) **False**   The amount required is 2–5 μg daily.
   (c) **True**   This explains the insidious onset of vitamin B_{12} deficiency.
   (d) **True**   This is classic pernicious anaemia and is associated with severe atrophic gastritis.
   (e) **False**   The site of absorption is the terminal ileum.

21 (a) **False**   More than 90% of food folate may be lost by heating.
   (b) **True**   Daily requirements are 100 μg, total body stores about 10 mg.
   (c) **False**   It is absorbed in the upper jejunum.
   (d) **False**   Serum folate is susceptible to minor changes in folic acid status. The red cell folate is more useful reflecting the level over the half-life of the red cells.
   (e) **True**   Due to increased cell turnover.

22 (a) **True**   Both haematinics are necessary for DNA synthesis. Lack causes defective nuclear maturation resulting in the production of large cells with an open nuclear chromatin meshwork, and ineffective erythropoiesis.
   (b) **False**   The most rapidly dividing cells are those of the alimentary tract and haemopoietic system; both are severely affected.
   (c) **False**   There is no satisfactory evidence that folic acid is required for the integrity of the nervous system. Reports of associated neuropathy have proved to be related to alcoholism or malignancy.
   (d) **True**   Vitamin B_{12} is essential for the maintenance of the myelin sheath. Deficiency can cause a peripheral neuropathy and later, subacute combined degeneration of the spinal cord.
   (e) **False**   Brain function is altered as evidenced by change of mood. Optic atrophy occasionally develops.

23 (a) **True**   The most common cause of a macrocytosis, usually with a normal haemoglobin concentration.
   (b) **True**   A brisk reticulocyte response will increase the MCV whether due to haemorrhage or haemolysis.
   (c) **True**   A macrocytosis is common.
   (d) **True**   Macrocytes can occur in many bone marrow infiltrations.
   (e) **False**   There is no evidence of a pancytopenia.

24 (a) **True**   The drug inhibits the ribonucleotide reductase enzyme system thus blocking DNA synthesis.
   (b) **True**   AZT mimics the thymine substrate required for DNA synthesis.
   (c) **False**   A slight increase in MCV occurs but rarely is sufficient to cause macrocytosis.
   (d) **True**   It is a folic acid antagonist.
   (e) **False**   This drug has no affect on red cell maturation.

25 Common features in anaemias due to vitamin B_{12} and folic acid deficiency are:
  (a) Oval macrocytosis in the peripheral blood film.
  (b) Hyperplastic erythropoiesis in the bone marrow.
  (c) Pancytopenia.
  (d) Hypersegmented neutrophils present in the peripheral blood.
  (e) Masking of the macrocytic blood appearances if concomitant iron deficiency exists.

26 In pernicious anaemia (PA):
  (a) The patient may present with a haemoglobin as low as 3–4 g/dl.
  (b) Blood transfusion should be avoided in patients presenting with a low haemoglobin concentration.
  (c) Patients may present with neurological manifestations but without anaemia.
  (d) The glossitis is due to coexisting iron deficiency.
  (e) Gastrointestinal symptoms are usually due to associated gut malignancy.

27 The following are related to the diagnosis of pernicious anaemia (PA):
  (a) A low serum B_{12} indicates a diagnosis of PA.
  (b) A patient with megaloblastic anaemia and a low B_{12} must have PA.
  (c) The red cell folate is low in 60% of patients.
  (d) A low radioactive vitamin B_{12} excretion in the urine (Schilling test) uncorrected by the oral administration of intrinsic factor (IF) is usual.
  (e) The presence of intrinsic factor antibodies is essential to confirm the diagnosis.

25 (a) **True**   The large red cells are the product of megaloblastic erythropoiesis.

(b) **True**   Despite the degree of hypercellularity, erythropoiesis is largely ineffective and the majority of cells formed are destroyed within the marrow.

(c) **False**   Both granulopoiesis and thrombopoiesis are also abnormal and ineffective.

(d) **True**   They are characteristic findings but occasionally they may also be found in iron deficiency anaemia and renal failure.

(e) **True**   Careful examination of the blood films shows some dimorphic changes (i.e. macrocytes and microcytes) and hypersegmented neutrophils.

26 (a) **True**   Some patients appear to be well-compensated at this level but increasing dyspnoea on exertion and angina are common symptoms.

(b) **True**   Blood transfusion can cause death due to circulatory overload. Parenteral vitamin B_{12} therapy is required.

(c) **True**   Sometimes myelin is affected before any marked changes in erythropoiesis occur.

(d) **False**   It is due to megaloblastic changes in the epithelial cells.

(e) **False**   Two-thirds of patients with PA have gastrointestinal symptoms, one of the most common of which is diarrhoea. The incidence of carcinoma of the stomach is, however, increased three-fold in this condition.

27 (a) **False**   There are other causes of a low serum B_{12}, including nutritional deficiency (vegans) and other causes of malabsorption both gastric and intestinal.

(b) **False**   As for (a). A low vitamin B_{12} may sometimes be found secondary to folate deficiency.

(c) **True**   This is due to trapping of methyltetrahydrofolate in the plasma as vitamin B_{12} is required for transfer of folate into red cell precursors.

(d) **False**   This result suggests malabsorption of the B_{12}/IF complex in the terminal ileum.

(e) **False**   These are found in the serum of 55% of patients.

28 These statements concern the diagnosis of folic acid deficiency:
  (a) Low serum and red cell folate concentrations always indicate folate deficiency.
  (b) A reticulocyte response following folic acid therapy confirms the diagnosis.
  (c) Suboptimal response to folate therapy may be due to co-existing infection.
  (d) A higher red cell folate concentration may occur in folate deficiency following a blood transfusion.
  (e) Tests to exclude malabsorption are essential in all folic acid deficient patients.

29 The following may produce megaloblastic anaemia:
  (a) Phenytoin.
  (b) Lead poisoning.
  (c) Trimethoprim.
  (d) Folinic acid.
  (e) Pyrimethamine.

30 Following initial treatment with parenteral vitamin B_{12} in pernicious anaemia:
  (a) The gastric atrophy is reversed.
  (b) The glossitis improves over 2–3 weeks.
  (c) The symptoms of subacute combined degeneration of the cord are markedly improved by the second week of treatment.
  (d) A peak reticulocyte response occurs 9–10 days after the start of therapy.
  (e) Marrow erythropoiesis becomes normoblastic within 24–48 h of treatment.

28 (a) **False**   Both levels are occasionally low in patients with pernicious anaemia, although high serum folates are usual in this condition. The diagnosis of folate deficiency often relies on excluding B_{12} deficiency.

(b) **False**   Some patients with B_{12} deficiency will respond to pharmacological doses of folic acid albeit briefly. Ideally folic acid should be given in physiological doses to confirm the diagnosis but this is rarely carried out in clinical practice.

(c) **True**   As may also occur with underlying malignancy, inflammatory disease or renal disease.

(d) **True**   The transfused cells contain normal amounts of folate. Always take blood samples for analysis before transfusion.

(e) **False**   Frequent causes are dietary lack, alcoholism, antifolate drugs or conditions of increasing folate demand (e.g. pregnancy or haemolysis). These conditions are often apparent from the clinical history and examination. Malabsorption syndromes need be sought only if the clinical features are suggestive or if the cause is unclear.

29 (a) **True**   In 50% of epileptic patients on long-term treatment both serum and red cell folate are low. Megaloblastic changes and macrocytosis are common. The mechanism is unclear.

(b) **False**   Lead produces a mild anaemia with a reduced red cell life span. Basophilic stippling of the red cells is common.

(c) **True**   Trimethoprim is a weak folate antagonist. It can precipitate folate deficiency but only when folate status is already marginal.

(d) **False**   It is a tetrahydrofolate.

(e) **True**   In the dose given for malaria prophylaxis it is unlikely but can develop with the higher dose used for the treatment of toxoplasmosis.

30 (a) **False**   It is due to autoimmune damage and persists.

(b) **True**   This represents the regeneration time of epithelium following the resumption of normal DNA synthesis.

(c) **False**   Recovery is slow and incomplete but improvement may continue for several months after commencing therapy. Demyelination stops when treatment begins.

(d) **False**   The peak response should be on the fifth to seventh day after treatment (assuming the day of therapy to be zero) following 100 μg hydroxocobalamin. This therapeutic trial can confirm the diagnosis. A further 5 mg given over the ensuing 2 weeks replenishes the body stores.

(e) **True**   Giant metamyelocytes persist, however, for some days because even with vitamin B_{12} they cannot develop.

31 A 75-year-old woman was admitted to hospital with a haemoglobin concentration of 3.2 g/l. She was confused and complained that she felt as though she was 'walking on cotton wool'. On examination she had glossitis, a raised jugular venous pressure, peripheral oedema and crepitations at both lung bases. The patient was treated with the appropriate haematinic and diuretics. Twelve hours after the start of treatment the patient complained of generalised weakness and collapsed. Among the investigations carried out was an ECG, which showed prominent U-waves. The patient recovered with further treatment and the following day was mentally alert and feeling better. She had an optimal response to the haematinic but after 2 weeks the haemoglobin stopped rising.
   (a) Folic acid was the appropriate haematinic for this patient.
   (b) A transfusion of whole blood should have been given.
   (c) The patient's ECG changes were probably due to hypokalaemia.
   (d) The rapid improvement in the patient's mental state is unusual.
   (e) The failure of the haemoglobin to increase at 2 weeks could be due to an associated iron deficiency.

32 The following statements relate to intravascular haemolysis:
   (a) Due to the high molecular weight of haemoglobin tetramers (64 500 daltons) haemoglobin rarely appears in the urine during an episode of intravascular haemolysis.
   (b) Red cells may show the 'bite' abnormality.
   (c) Plasma haptoglobins are low.
   (d) Methaemalbuminaemia can occur.
   (e) Iron may be found in the urine.

33 Microangiopathic haemolytic anaemia (MAHA) is a fragmentation anaemia secondary to abnormalities of the microvasculature and is found in the following:
   (a) Haemolytic uraemic syndrome.
   (b) Meningococcal meningitis without bacteraemia.
   (c) March haemoglobinuria.
   (d) Thrombotic thrombocytopenic purpura.
   (e) Prosthetic heart valve haemolysis.

31 (a) **False** The most likely diagnosis is vitamin B_{12} deficiency. Administration of folate may precipitate further neurological damage. When there is urgency both haematinics can be given at the same time.

(b) **False** This is very dangerous if there is heart failure. If deemed life saving, one unit of packed red cells can be given slowly with a diuretic.

(c) **True** This can be a cause of sudden death early in treatment due to increased demand for potassium in cell turnover. The plasma K^+ should always be measured and supplements given if low or if diuretics are used.

(d) **False** Subjective and objective improvement often occurs during the first 24 h of treatment.

(e) **True** Although the marrow iron stores are unusually high in megalo-blastic anaemia, they can be depleted by excessive demand for iron associated with resumption of normal erythropoiesis.

32 (a) **False** Free haemoglobin in the plasma is dissociated into dimers of approximately 32 000 daltons which pass into the renal tubules and may exceed the tubular absorptive capacity.

(b) **True** Intravascular haemolysis due to oxidative red cell damage will cause red cell membrane change and the creation of aggregated denatured haemoglobin (Heinz bodies). Some cells are destroyed within the circulation whilst removal of Heinz bodies by the splenic macrophages results in a red cell that appears to have a bite taken out of it.

(c) **True** Free plasma haemoglobin is bound by haptoglobins to an amount of 125 mg haemoglobin/dl of plasma. These complexes are rapidly removed by the liver and plasma haptoglobin may be depleted.

(d) **True** Usually in acute haemolysis. Treatment of plasma with a strong reducing agent (Schumm's test) reveals a characteristic haemochromogen spectroscopic band.

(e) **True** Some of the haemoglobin filtered by the renal glomeruli is taken up by the tubular cells where the iron is stored as haemosiderin. Subsequent desquamation of the tubular cells results in haemosiderinuria.

33 (a) **True** A syndrome usually found in childhood characterised by MAHA, thrombocytopenia and renal failure. There appears to be an abnor-mal interaction between the patient's platelets and glomerular endothelium.

(b) **False** Meningitis *per se* will not cause disseminated intravascular coagu-lation (DIC) and MAHA. Once there is septicaemia, microthrombus formation and endotoxic damage to the microvasculature occur, with fragmentation of red cells in the peripheral blood.

(c) **False** This follows walking or running on a hard surface. Red cells are damaged in the superficial vessels of the feet but the blood film appearances are normal and there are no fragments.

(d) **True** A disease usually occurring in adults comprising fever, anaemia, thrombocytopenia, renal failure and fluctuating neurological signs.

(e) **False** Haemolysis occurs due to red cell trauma at the valve interface or due to a periprosthetic leak with turbulence. There is no defect of the microvasculature.

34 Which of the following are associated with intravascular haemolysis?
   (a) Dapsone.
   (b) Paroxysmal nocturnal haemoglobinuria.
   (c) Pyruvate kinase deficiency.
   (d) Idiopathic warm-type autoimmune haemolytic anaemia.
   (e) Hereditary spherocytosis.

35 The following concern extravascular haemolysis of red cells:
   (a) Conjugated bilirubin in the plasma is increased.
   (b) Urinary urobilinogen is increased.
   (c) Destruction of the red cells occurs primarily in the liver.
   (d) It is characterised by the passage of dark urine.
   (e) A normal serum bilirubin precludes the diagnosis of haemolysis.

36 The following are statements about the haematological findings in haemolytic
   anaemia:
   (a) The reticulocyte count is usually increased.
   (b) The ratio of myeloid to erythroid cells in bone marrow is normal.
   (c) The development of a pancytopenia may be due to associated folic acid
       deficiency.
   (d) A chromium-labelled red cell half-life ($t_{\frac{1}{2}}$) of 27 days.
   (e) Erythropoiesis may be macronormoblastic.

37 The following statements concern clinical features secondary to haemolysis:
   (a) The patient may not be anaemic.
   (b) Clinically detectable jaundice is usually apparent if the plasma bilirubin
       exceeds 20 μmol/l.
   (c) X-ray changes in the bones of patients with acquired haemolytic anaemia are
       very common.
   (d) Splenomegaly is a characteristic feature.
   (e) Biliary colic may occur.

34 (a) **True** The administration of an oxidant drug, particularly to a patient with impairment of the pentose phosphate pathway caused by G-6-PD deficiency will often lead to a failure of the red cell redox system resulting in acute lysis.

(b) **True** A clonal disorder in which red cells are susceptible to complement mediated lysis with resultant haemoglobinaemia and haemoglobinuria.

(c) **False** Haemolysis is predominantly extravascular due to energy requirements exceeding ATP formation.

(d) **False** IgG anti-red cell antibodies bind to the red cells. This abnormality is recognized by the Fc-receptor of splenic macrophages with subsequent phagocytosis. Partial phagocytosis results in spherocytosis.

(e) **False** Extravascular haemolysis is characteristic.

35 (a) **False** The bilirubin is unconjugated and bound to albumin.

(b) **True** The total amount of bilirubin conjugated in the liver is increased but this is easily excreted via the bowel. The increased quantity of gut urobilinogen results in a greater reabsorption and urinary excretion.

(c) **False** Although destruction occurs within the whole reticuloendothelial system, the spleen is usually the predominant site.

(d) **False** Bilirubin is not found in the urine (acholuric jaundice). Urinary urobilinogen increases and the urine often darkens on standing due to urobilin formation.

(e) **False** Although commonly in the range of 20–60 μmol/l, the serum bilirubin may be normal.

36 (a) **True** Due to increased erythropoietic activity and a reduced marrow transit time. Circulating nucleated red cells may also be found.

(b) **False** Due to erythroid hyperplasia the normal myeloid/erythroid ratio is reduced from about 3–4:1 to 1:1 or less.

(c) **True** Folate requirements are increased due to the high red cell turnover and megaloblastic changes develop. Oral folic acid supplements are usually given in chronic haemolytic states. Severe folate lack can sometimes precipitate an aplastic crisis.

(d) **False** Although the normal red cell life is 100–120 days ($t^{\frac{1}{2}}$ = 50–60 days), using chromium-labelled cells the normal $t^{\frac{1}{2}}$ is, for various technical reasons, 25–32 days. In haemolytic anaemia the $t^{\frac{1}{2}}$ may be much shorter than this.

(e) **True** The developing nucleated red cells are larger than usual. This reflects a compensatory increase in the rate of erythroid turnover.

37 (a) **True** Due to compensatory erythroid hyperplasia the red cell survival is often less than 20 days before anaemia develops.

(b) **False** Values in excess of 40 μmol/l are required to produce discernible icterus of the sclerae.

(c) **False** The typical hair-on-end appearance of the skull due to widening of the diploic space and expanded medulla of the long bones is usually seen only in the severe thalassaemic syndromes, sickle- cell disease and other severe chronic haemolytic anaemias.

(d) **True** Due to hyperplasia, as it is the major site of red cell destruction.

(e) **True** Due to increased bilirubin excretion in the bile, gallstones may develop in any chronic haemolytic anaemia.

38 The following statements concern hereditary spherocytosis:
   (a) Haemolytic crises may be precipitated by intercurrent infection.
   (b) The osmotic fragility of the red cells is usually abnormal.
   (c) Spherocytes are usually detectable in the peripheral blood at birth.
   (d) Clinical remission following splenectomy is due to a marked reduction in the numbers of circulating spherocytes.
   (e) Splenectomy in children is accompanied by an increased risk of severe infection.

39 Which of the following mechanisms underly the thalassaemia syndromes?
   (a) Nonsense mutations.
   (b) Frame shifts.
   (c) Gene deletion.
   (d) Failure of DNA transcription.
   (e) Failure of RNA splicing.

40 The following statements concern the haematological findings in untreated β^0-thalassemia major:
   (a) Haemoglobin F is virtually the only haemoglobin present.
   (b) Target cells are common.
   (c) Nucleated red cells are common.
   (d) The white cell count is usually normal.
   (e) 50% of the red cells contain Howell–Jolly bodies.

38 (a) **True** Infection commonly results in intermittent exacerbation of haemolysis, although erythroblastopenia due to parvovirus may occur.

(b) **True** Occasionally only 1–2% of the circulating cells are spherocytic; this will not be detected by the osmotic fragility test.

(c) **True** Spherocytes are present at birth and may cause neonatal jaundice usually on the second or third day after delivery.

(d) **False** The spherocytes persist but are no longer selectively trapped and destroyed within the spleen. An approximately normal red cell life-span is found postoperatively.

(e) **True** The spleen appears to be important in limiting infection caused by Gram-positive bacteria in children. Pneumococcal septicaemia can be minimised by the administration of polyvalent pneumococcal vaccine and long-term penicillin.

39 (a) **True** Nonsense mutations usually involve a single nucleotide producing a new stop codon, which terminates the translation of mRNA prematurely.

(b) **True** One or more deletions or insertions can produce a stop codon downstream and alter the translation of mRNA with the same effect as (a) above.

(c) **True** Gene deletion is common in alpha thalassaemia and occurs in some beta thalassaemias. In the former, either of the two gene sites on each chromosome 16 can be deleted, giving a range of phenotypes from the asymptomatic carrier state to fatal hydrops fetalis.

(d) **True** Changes in promotor sequences, usually by single base substitutions, lead to reduced mRNA production.

(e) **True** Changes in bases at the junction of introns and exons disrupt the normal splicing mechanism essential for mRNA translation to normal protein.

40 (a) **True** This is the most severe form of thalassemia with no chain production. Haemoglobin electrophoresis reveals a haemoglobin of 98% with a haemoglobin A_2 of 2%. In $^+$ thalassemia there is some chain production with up to 20% haemoglobin A present.

(b) **True** The prominent feature in the blood film, which also shows gross hypochromia together with aniso- and poikilocytosis.

(c) **True** Especially in those patients with the lowest haemoglobin.

(d) **False** Often raised (15–30 × 10^9/l) and appears higher unless the nucleated red cell count is subtracted.

(e) **False** Howell–Jolly bodies, which are small, rounded nuclear remnants, are only prominent after splenectomy.

41 The following are statements concerning beta thalassemia major:
   (a) Iron overload is the major cause of death.
   (b) Severe anaemia occurs in the neonatal period.
   (c) Gross hepatosplenomegaly is common.
   (d) There is often evidence of endocrine disease.
   (e) A pancytopenia may develop.

42 The following statements concern sickle cell anaemia (HbSS):
   (a) The haemoglobin concentration is commonly 6–9 g/dl.
   (b) The higher the proportion of haemoglobin F the worse the clinical condition.
   (c) Patients are protected from the effects of *Plasmodium falciparum* infection.
   (d) Reticulocytopenia may suddenly occur.
   (e) Sufferers easily become dehydrated.

41 (a) **True**   Sudden death due to cardiac failure is a common terminal event. It is due to anaemia and iron deposition in cardiac muscle caused by excessive iron absorption and regular transfusions.

  (b) **False**   At birth infants with beta thalassaemia major are not anaemic; this develops as globin gene switching takes place.

  (c) **True**   Due to hyperplasia of the reticuloendothelial tissue, extramedullary haemopoiesis and cirrhosis with portal hypertension due to iron deposition.

  (d) **True**   Failure to develop secondary sexual characteristics, diabetes mellitus and adrenal insufficiency can occur due to iron deposition in the endocrine glands.

  (e) **True**   Due to splenic sequestration (hypersplenism) or, less commonly, an aplastic crisis.

42 (a) **True**   Despite the anaemia, in 'steady state' conditions symptoms of anaemia are not severe due to the usual compensatory mechanisms and a marked right shift in the oxygen dissociation curve.

  (b) **False**   The presence of any other haemoglobin form (especially HbA and F) interferes with the aggregation of deoxygenated HbS molecules and minimises sickling with resulting milder disease.

  (c) **False**   Malaria is a major cause of death in endemic areas. Patients with sickle cell trait have some measure of protection. This is due to the high oxygen consumption of the malarial parasites, which induces sickling. Splenic sequestration of the sickle cells occurs and destruction of the parasites follows.

  (d) **True**   Bone marrow failure may occur suddenly in association with infection often due to parvovirus. The condition may be compounded by folate deficiency.

  (e) **True**   There is an inability to concentrate the urine. Correction of dehydration is one of the mainstays of treatment during a crisis. The accompanying change in viscosity will worsen the existing obstruction to blood flow in the microcirculation.

43 The following are further statements concerning sickle cell anaemia (HbSS):
  (a) Infection is a major cause of death.
  (b) Pleural pain is a common complication.
  (c) Monthly transfusion is the mainstay of treatment.
  (d) Irregularities of finger length may occur.
  (e) Splenomegaly is common in adults.

44 The following are further statements relating to sickle cell anaemia (HbSS):
  (a) Cerebrovascular events are rare.
  (b) Treatment with hydroxyurea results in a dramatic clinical improvement.
  (c) Oral contraceptives are contraindicated.
  (d) The incidence of opiate drug dependency is high.
  (e) Sudden massive splenomegaly may occur.

43 (a) **True**   Especially in young children. Prompt treatment with antibiotics is an important aspect of treatment. Common infections are pneumococcal septicaemia and meningitis. Children should be given the appropriate vaccines and prophylactic penicillin. Infections will precipitate crises. These are usually accompanied by increased haemolysis.

   (b) **True**   Either due to infection or due to infarction due to local sickling. Ventilation/perfusion scanning usually shows multiple perfusion defects.

   (c) **False**   Regular transfusion has attendant risks and increases viscosity. Transfusion during crises may be necessary and if the haemoglobin becomes too low exchange transfusion may be indicated. This procedure may have some value in pregnancy and prior to surgery.

   (d) **True**   Due to microinfarction in the small bones of the hands and feet and subsequent uneven growth of the digits. This is termed hand/foot syndrome and can be very painful. Similarly, avascular necrosis of the femoral head can occur in teenagers.

   (e) **False**   Splenomegaly develops in infancy but becomes progressively reduced in size by vascular obstruction and subsequent infarction (autosplenectomy). Some patients with higher levels of haemoglobin F have fewer infarctive crises and retain splenomegaly into adulthood.

44 (a) **False**   Such events are not uncommon in children and once they happen, tend to be recurrent. These patients are often maintained on a hypertransfusion programme to suppress endogenous HbS production.

   (b) **False**   Several drugs have been used to stimulate haemoglobin F production as a strategy to reduce the severity of the disease. All have important side-effects and poor efficacy.

   (c) **False**   The thrombogenic risk of low-dose oestrogen contraceptives is low and any risk is far outweighed by a pregnancy either leading to term or termination.

   (d) **False**   Opiates are frequently necessary as microvascular infarctive episodes can be painful at any site. Patients are often not only in severe pain but frightened. Despite this, drug dependency occurs in only a minority of patients and may be due to other psychosocial problems.

   (e) **True**   In young children the liver and spleen may suddenly increase in size with pooling of red cells and acute anaemia (sequestration crisis).

45 The following concern glucose-6-phosphate dehydrogenase (G-6-PD) deficiency:
   (a) Females commonly have clinical symptoms.
   (b) It is the most common red cell enzyme deficiency to be found in clinical practice.
   (c) Neonatal jaundice resulting in kernicterus can occur.
   (d) Favism may produce profound anaemia.
   (e) Infection rarely precipitates haemolysis.

46 A 70-year-old man was seen in the haematology clinic. He complained of tiredness, passing red urine and of cold, discoloured fingers. On examination he was found to be pale and the spleen was just palpable. Investigations showed the haemoglobin to be 10.5 g/dl. Marked autoagglutination of the red cells was present in the blood film. Some spherocytes were present and the reticulocyte count was 180 × 10⁹/l. Microscopy of the urine showed that no intact red cells were present. Which of the following statements are correct?
   (a) The most likely diagnosis is cold haemagglutinin disease.
   (b) The direct antiglobulin (Coombs') test is likely to be positive.
   (c) Treatment with methyldopa could produce this haematological picture.
   (d) Symptomatic treatment is often all that is necessary in this condition.
   (e) An underlying lymphoma should be sought.

47 Anaesthetic complications can occur in the following haemoglobinopathies:
   (a) Homozygous sickle-cell disease.
   (b) Haemoglobin C disease.
   (c) Haemoglobin SC disease.
   (d) Haemoglobin E disease.
   (e) Sickle-cell β° thalassaemia.

45 (a) **False**   The gene is carried on the X chromosome and is therefore sex-linked. Females rarely have low enough G-6-PD concentrations to cause haemolysis unless they inherit two affected X-chromosomes.

(b) **True**   It is estimated that 100 million people carry the gene.

(c) **True**   There are many isoenzyme variants to be found in this condition; two of the most common occur in people of African origin and those from the Mediterranean. It is this latter variant in which neonatal jaundice and even kernicteris can occur.

(d) **True**   Hypersensitivity to broad beans does not occur in all patients with this deficiency but in those affected the haemoglobin concentration may fall below 4 g/dl.

(e) **False**   Apart from the ingestion of oxidant drugs, one of the most common causes of a mild haemolytic episode is intercurrent infection and fever.

46 (a) **True**   The history of cold discoloured fingers is highly suggestive of Raynaud's phenomenon or acrocyanosis. This together with probable haemoglobinuria and autoagglutination of the red cells points to a diagnosis of cold haemagglutinin disease (CHAD).

(b) **True**   The cause of haemolytic anaemia found in CHAD is the development of a monoclonal IgM antibody with anti-I specificity. The I antigen is found on adult red cells and its counterpart, i, on fetal red cells. Anti-I is a cold antibody that combines with the I antigen in the peripheral cooler parts of the body. This reaction involves the fixation of complement to the red cell membrane with subsequent red cell lysis. As the blood returns to the body 'core' temperature of 37°C, the anti-I dissociates itself from the antigen. If blood is taken and the red cells are separated at 37°C the Coombs' test will be positive but only complement will be found on the red cell surface. The antihuman globulin reagent used in the Coombs' test includes anti-C3 and anti-C4.

(c) **False**   Methyldopa causes the development of an IgG autoantibody with Rhesus blood group specificity. A warm autoimmune haemolytic anaemia (autoantibody active at 37°C) may rarely develop during treatment with methyldopa but most commonly it is characterised by a positive direct antiglobulin test with no evidence of haemolysis.

(d) **True**   Warmth and restricted outdoor activity in cold weather are often all that is required to prevent haemolytic episodes. Chlorambucil is sometimes effective in reducing the IgM paraprotein concentration with subsequent clinical improvement.

(e) **True**   About 10% of patients with CHAD develop a lymphoma but it may be present at the time of diagnosis.

47 (a) **True**   But the risks are low providing inadvertent hypoxia is avoided, adequate hydration maintained and any postoperative infections promptly treated. (With modern anaesthetic practice sickle-cell trait should never present an anaesthetic risk.)

(b) **False**   There are no added anaesthetic risks. Haemolysis in this condition is usually mild and the patients often asymptomatic.

(c) **True**   The proportion of haemoglobin S (50%) is greater than sickle cell trait (30–40%) — this increases the risk.

(d) **False**   As (b) above.

(e) **True**   Haemoglobin S comprises 80–95% of the total haemoglobin.

48 The following drugs are associated with the development of a positive direct
   antiglobulin test (DAGT) (direct Coombs' test):
   (a) High-dose penicillin.
   (b) Rifampicin.
   (c) Carbimazole.
   (d) Cephradine.
   (e) Chloramphenicol.

49 A British business man returns from Kenya to the UK and develops an intermittent
   temperature, which occurs on most evenings. Whilst abroad he took malarial
   chemoprophylaxis and was still taking this 6 days after his return when he
   presented to his general practitioner. A full blood count shows a 2% parasitaemia
   with occasional red cells containing two malarial ring forms. His haemoglobin is
   12.8 g/dl and white cell count 3.8 x 10^9/l, lymphocytes comprise 43% of the
   differential count and some are atypical. Which of the following are correct?
   (a) He should be told to continue chemoprophylaxis for a further 4 weeks.
   (b) The infection is most likely due to *Plasmodium vivax*.
   (c) The treatment of choice is quinine.
   (d) Treatment with primaquine is essential.
   (e) The atypical lymphocytes suggest a concomitant viral infection.

50 The following relate to the neutrophil granulocyte:
   (a) Neutrophil maturation occurs in the bone marrow.
   (b) The number of neutrophils counted in the peripheral blood represents the
       total blood granulocyte pool.
   (c) Neutrophils spend several days in the circulation.
   (d) The peripheral neutrophil count is increased during sustained exercise.
   (e) The neutrophil count does not rise for 2–3 days following an infection due to
       the slow generation time of granulocytes.

48 (a) **True**   Penicillin can bind to the surface of the red cells creating a potentially antigenic cell–hapten complex. Some individuals develop IgG antibodies to the complex with consequent extravascular haemolysis.

(b) **True**   This drug forms complexes with plasma proteins becoming antigenic. When the drug is reintroduced immune complexes are formed which link with the red cell membrane and activate the complement sequence (the so-called innocent bystander reaction).

(c) **False**   Neutropenia is the most serious unwanted effect.

(d) **True**   Cephradine acts much in the same way as penicillin but may modify some red cell proteins and produce a positive DAGT.

(e) **False**   Chloramphenicol may produce an aplastic anaemia. The risk is probably 1:60 000.

49 (a) **False**   The patient clearly has malaria and should be treated. Prophylaxis is not absolute and breakthrough can occur.

(b) **False**   The temperature sequence is not that of *P. vivax* or *P. ovale*, i.e. tertian — a temperature every other day (a three-day pattern) or *P. malariae*, i.e. quartan — a temperature every third day (a four-day pattern). In addition there is a moderate parasitaemia with multiple infection of the red cells. Finally the patient has visited an area where chloroquine resistant strains of *P. falciparum* occur.

(c) **True**   Unless there is good reason to suggest that a patient has acquired malaria in an area where chloroquine resistance is unknown, quinine must be the first line treatment. It can be given orally or intravenously depending upon the severity of the illness. If in doubt always seek advice from a specialist centre.

(d) **False**   Primaquine is given with chloroquine for the treatment of all benign malarias. It is not required for the treatment of *P. falciparum*.

(e) **False**   Atypical lymphocytes are commonly found in malarial infections. Their presence in the absence of parasites in the blood film should raise a suspicion that the patient may well have malaria and that further blood samples should be taken during a febrile stage.

50 (a) **True**   In the adult, maturation takes about 10 days.

(b) **False**   Half of the total blood granulocyte pool is marginated on the endothelial surface of the blood vessels. Only granulocytes in the circulating pool are measured by blood sampling.

(c) **False**   The time spent in the circulation (blood transit time) is short with a $t\frac{1}{2}$ of 6–8 hours.

(d) **True**   Due to marginated neutrophils entering the circulating pool (demargination).

(e) **False**   In addition to the mitotic pool of neutrophil precursor cells in the marrow, there is a large storage pool of neutrophils, at least ten times the total blood granulocyte pool, which is readily available when required. Some of these cells are not completely mature as shown by the 'left shift' (i.e. increased numbers of bilobed neutrophils and occasional metamyelocytes) seen in response to infection.

51 The following concern a peripheral blood neutrophil leucocytosis:
    (a) If neutrophils comprise 80% of a total white cell count of $8 \times 10^9/l$, then, by definition, a neutrophil leucocytosis exists.
    (b) It is commonly caused by an acute pyogenic infection.
    (c) A postoperative increase in neutrophils is a reliable indication of associated infection.
    (d) It often follows severe haemorrhage.
    (e) It is a feature of myeloproliferative disorders.

52 The following statements relate to GM-CSF (granulocyte/macrophage colony stimulating factor):
    (a) It is a soluble factor that can modify the behaviour and growth pattern of cells.
    (b) It causes marked thrombocytosis.
    (c) It can be administered in pharmacological doses to shorten the period of neutropenia following cytotoxic therapy.
    (d) It can be used to treat the anaemia of renal failure.
    (e) It will elevate the neutrophil count in neutropenic patients infected with HIV (human immunodeficiency virus).

53 The following statements concern lymphocytes:
    (a) Lymphocytes are derived from pluripotent stem cells in the thymus.
    (b) T lymphocytes are present in the paracortical areas of lymph nodes.
    (c) T lymphocytes are the principal source of immunoglobulins.
    (d) B lymphocyte activity is modulated by T lymphocytes.
    (e) B lymphocytes are responsible for immunity to *Pneumocystis carinii*.

51 (a) **False** The absolute neutrophil count in this example is $6.4 \times 10^9/l$, an absolute neutrophil leucocytosis is defined as a count exceeding $7.5 \times 10^9/l$.

(b) **True** Although Gram-positive and Gram-negative pyogenic cocci are the most common causes, a similar response will occur to infections due to Gram-negative bacilli of gut origin.

(c) **False** Any tissue damage (including surgical operations) will cause a neutrophil leucocytosis. Fractures, crush inquiries, burns, malignancy and ischaemia, including myocardial infarction, are other examples of tissue damage that result in a neutrophil leucocytosis.

(d) **True** Haemorrhage and haemolysis result in marrow proliferation and a neutrophil leucocytosis and thrombocytosis may occur in addition to the increase in reticulocytes (red cells that have recently entered the peripheral blood from the marrow).

(e) **True** Autonomous myeloid proliferation, as opposed to reactive, is the other major mechanism by which a neutrophil leucocytosis may result.

52 (a) **True** This is the definition of a cytokine. Other cytokines include the other colony stimulating factors (including erythropoietin), the interleukins, the interferons and the tumour necrosis factors.

(b) **False** An increase in the platelet count is not seen in humans following administration of GM-CSF.

(c) **True** The ability to shorten the duration of cytotoxic-induced neutropenia may result in a decreased susceptibility to infection in patients undergoing cytotoxic therapy for malignant tumours. In addition, the more rapid recovery of the marrow may permit higher doses of cytotoxic drugs to be administered.

(d) **False** GM-CSF is not an erythroid growth factor. The anaemia of renal failure will often respond to the administration of erythropoietin.

(e) **True** The primary immunodeficiency in AIDS is lymphopenia affecting predominantly CD4-positive helper lymphocytes. Some patients eventually develop neutropenia, which may result from autoimmune destruction or bone marrow insufficiency resulting from infection of neutrophil precursors by HIV or the result of antiviral therapy such as AZT. GM-CSF has been shown to increase neutrophil counts in AIDS patients with inadequate marrow production of neutrophils.

53 (a) **False** Lymphocytes appear to be derived from the pluripotent stem cells that also give rise to myeloid (bone marrow) cells. Proliferation and maturation of lymphocytes occurs at many sites including bone marrow, thymus, spleen and lymph nodes.

(b) **True** T cell development takes place in the thymus and once mature, T cells circulate in the blood before localising in the major T cell region (paracortex) of lymph nodes.

(c) **False** Plasma cells are terminally differentiated B cells that secrete immunoglobulins.

(d) **True** T cells can either enhance or suppress B cell function.

(e) **False** T cell immunity (cellular immunity) is required to prevent pneumocystis infection

54 An absolute lymphocytosis (lymphocyte count $> 4.0 \times 10^9/l$) usually occurs in the following conditions:
   (a) *Bordetella pertussis* infection.
   (b) Tuberculosis.
   (c) During the prodromal phase of 'viral' hepatitis A.
   (d) Chronic lymphocytic leukaemia.
   (e) Polyarteritis nodosa.

55 Which of the following clinical features or circumstances might be associated with these results? WBC $10.8 \times 10^9/l$; differential count: neutrophils 60%, lymphocytes 27%, monocytes 2%, eosinophils 11%:
   (a) Mediastinal lymph node enlargement.
   (b) *Entamoeba coli* infection.
   (c) Ampicillin therapy.
   (d) Pemphigus.
   (e) Allergic rhinitis.

56 The following statements concern infectious mononucleosis:
   (a) The disease is associated with the presence of the Epstein–Barr virus (EBV).
   (b) It is highly contagious.
   (c) The most constant symptom is a sore throat.
   (d) Palpable splenomegaly is frequently evident.
   (e) Ampicillin has a beneficial effect on the sore throat.

54 (a) **True**   Lymphocyte counts of 20 × 10⁹/l or higher are common, especially in children.

  (b) **False**   Tuberculosis and other chronic bacterial diseases can produce a relative lymphocytosis. The distinction between absolute and relative counts must be fully appreciated. A long search to reveal the cause of a relative lymphocytosis is often fruitless whereas the significance of the absolute neutropenia which accompanies it is ignored.

  (c) **False**   It is usually associated with a neutropenia and relative lymphocytosis. Later in the disease there may be an increase in lymphocytes which are morphologically atypical.

  (d) **True**   Often the diagnosis is clear from the typical blood picture. In the middle-aged and elderly a persistent mild lymphocytosis of unknown origin should be observed and its evolution monitored.

  (e) **False**   A neutrophil leucocytosis and, often an eosinophilia, are the characteristic white cell abnormalities in this condition.

55 (a) **True**   The presence of a mild to moderate eosinophilia with mediastinal lymphadenopathy is highly suggestive of Hodgkin's disease.

  (b) **False**   This is a non-pathogenic protozoon. Invasive *Entamoeba histolytica* may be associated with eosinophilia. Stool examination for parasites, e.g. ascaris, toxocara and hookworm may be necessary to elucidate the cause of eosinophilia.

  (c) **True**   Drug hypersensitivity is a common cause of eosinophilia in the UK.

  (d) **True**   Many skin disorders, especially those of an allergic nature are associated with eosinophilia.

  (e) **True**   Allergic reactions are the most common cause of eosinophilia in the Western world.

56 (a) **True**   Infectious mononucleosis is usually an acute illness caused by primary infection with EBV.

  (b) **False**   Infectivity is very low. Intimate oral contact is thought to be a common mode of transfer.

  (c) **True**   Pharyngitis together with fever and cervical lymphadenopathy constitute the clinical triad in this condition.

  (d) **True**   The spleen is usually tender and enlarged 3–5 cm below the left midcostal margin.

  (e) **False**   Ampicillin will, however, precipitate a maculopapular rash in many patients. It should not be given to patients suspected of having infectious mononucleosis.

57 The following features relate to infectious mononucleosis:
  (a) There is a T cell lymphocytosis during the first week of the illness.
  (b) High titre antisheep red cell antibodies are present in the serum.
  (c) Liver function tests are usually abnormal.
  (d) Antibody production is generally depressed.
  (e) Recurrent infection is common.

58 A 12-year-old presents with a mild sore throat and fever of 4 days' duration. Examination reveals posterior cervical lymphadenopathy and a fading maculopapular
   rash. The peripheral white count is $5.0 \times 10^9/l$; 60% are lymphocytes, many of
   which are atypical. The monospot test is negative. The following statements are
   true or false?
  (a) The patient has an absolute lymphocytosis.
  (b) The infectious mononucleosis (IM) screening test should be repeated in 1
      week.
  (c) A history of contact with an individual suffering from rubella is relevant.
  (d) Cytomegalovirus infection (CMV) could cause these findings.
  (e) A history of contact with cats could be important.

57 (a) **False**   A mild neutropenia or neutrophilia may be seen in the first week. Subsequently there is a T cell proliferative response to EBV-infected B cells. Thus most of the 'atypical' lymphocytes with large nuclei and abundant basophilic, often vacuolated, cytoplasm are reactive T cells.

  (b) **True**   These are the heterophile antibodies, which also agglutinate horse and ox cells. Heterophile antibody is antibody that binds antigen unrelated to the antigen that stimulated its production. Heterophile antibodies may be present in normal serum and occur in a variety of pathological conditions but a rising titre of heterophile antibody which is adsorbed by ox cells but not guinea-pig kidney is consistent with the diagnosis of infectious mononucleosis. This is the basis of the traditional Paul–Bunnell test, which is now rarely performed as there are several rapid commercial kits available.

  (c) **True**   Serum liver transaminase levels are elevated in more than 90% of patients. The liver is sometimes palpable but clinical jaundice is uncommon.

  (d) **False**   Serum IgM, and to a lesser extent IgG, concentrations are increased. Autoantibody production may occur resulting in an autoimmune haemolytic anaemia or thrombocytopenia.

  (e) **False**   A recurrence is extremely rare.

58 (a) **False**   The absolute lymphocyte count is $3.0 \times 10^9/l$. The normal upper limit is $3.5 \times 10^9/l$.

  (b) **True**   The screening test is commonly positive in infectious mononucleosis by the end of the first week of the illness but it may be delayed to the second or third week. The Paul–Bunnell can remain negative in 50% of childhood cases and 10% of adult cases.

  (c) **True**   Rubella could cause this clinical picture. However, case-to-case spread of clinical illness seldom occurs.

  (d) **True**   If the screening test remains negative, CMV may be the cause of all of these findings, although cervical lymphadenopathy is not as common in this condition as it is in infectious mononucleosis. The diagnosis may be confirmed by a rising antibody titre to cytomegalovirus but peak titres may not occur until 4–6 weeks after the onset of symptoms.

  (e) **True**   Toxoplasmosis is another cause of Paul–Bunnell-negative infectious mononucleosis fever syndrome. Cats are thought to be a common reservoir of infection. Oocysts excreted by cats can remain infective in moist soil for months and contact with contaminated soil can be more important than direct contact with cats. Diagnosis may be confirmed by a rising titre in the Sabin–Feldman dye test, which detects IgG antibody though toxoplasma-specific IgM antibody; indirect immunofluorescence and enzyme-linked immunosorbent assay (ELISA), are increasingly used.

59 The following are typical peripheral blood abnormalities found in acquired immune deficiency syndrome:
   (a) Monocytopenia.
   (b) Reticulocytosis.
   (c) Lymphopenia.
   (d) Granulocytic 'left shift'.
   (e) Spherocytosis.

60 Clinical aspects of HIV infection include:
   (a) Acute infection can produce an infectious mononucleosis-like syndrome.
   (b) Antibodies to HIV are detectable 14 days after infection.
   (c) The development of persistent generalised lymphadenopathy (PGL) indicates the development of acquired immunodeficiency syndrome (AIDS).
   (d) Opportunistic infection of the central nervous system.
   (e) Patients with Kaposi's sarcoma have a better prognosis than those with opportunistic infections.

61 The following conditions occurring in an individual infected with HIV indicate the development of AIDS:
   (a) Thrombocytopenia.
   (b) Persistent fever for 6 weeks.
   (c) Peripheral neuropathy.
   (d) Ophthalmic herpes zoster.
   (e) Primary lymphoma of the brain.

59 (a) **True**   A reduction in a monocyte count occurs in up to 40% of patients.

(b) **False**   Reticulocytopenia is the rule. It is associated with anaemia secondary to underlying infection or inflammation or megaloblastoid dyserythropoiesis.

(c) **True**   A deficiency of CD4-positive lymphocytes is the primary cause of the immunodeficiency syndrome.

(d) **True**   Band forms, metamyelocytes and myelocytes occur either due to infection or myeloid dysplasia.

(e) **False**   Spherocytosis is uncommon as haemolysis secondary to autoantibody production is unusual.

60 (a) **True**   Acute infection may cause fever, sweats, malaise, anorexia nervosa, myalgia, headache, sore throat, diarrhoea, a macular rash and generalised lymphadenopathy. Acute infection may however be asymptomatic.

(b) **False**   Seroconversion generally takes 3–8 weeks. Within this time patients are infectious.

(c) **False**   Most patients with PGL are asymptomatic and the majority do not develop AIDS in the subsequent 12 months.

(d) **True**   Many opportunistic infections occur in patients with AIDS and these may involve the CNS. In particular *Toxoplasma gondii* may cause mass lesions in the brain, cytomegalovirus may cause a meningoencephalitis and cryptococcus can cause meningitis.

(e) **True**   Patients seldom die as a result of the tumour. Localised lesions respond to radiotherapy whilst advanced disease may respond to antiviral therapy, combination cytotoxic therapy or intra-lesional interferon.

61 (a) **False**   Haematological manifestations may occur long before the patient is severely immunodeficient. Anaemia and neutropenia may also occur.

(b) **False**   Fever or diarrhoea for more than 1 month or weight loss in excess of 10% represent constitutional disease, but not AIDS.

(c) **False**   Painful sensory neuropathy indicates neurological disease. Other neurological disorders include dementia, aseptic meningitis and myelopathy. Dementia is considered as part of the AIDS syndrome.

(d) **False**   Reactivation of herpes zoster involving one dermatome is common but only multidermatomal zoster is considered indicative of AIDS.

(e) **True**   Approximately 5% of patients with AIDS develop non-Hodgkin's lymphoma. They are mainly of B cell origin, characterised by extranodal involvement and poor response to cytotoxic therapy. They often involve the CNS, bone marrow, bowel, oropharynx and rectum.

62 The following are statements relating to chromosomal analysis in haematological malignancies:
   (a) Chromosomes are visible only in the condensed form which they adopt at metaphase during cell division.
   (b) Each chromosome has arms of unequal length.
   (c) A translocation results in loss of a chromosome.
   (d) All acquired chromosome abnormalities result from clonal proliferation.
   (e) Chromosomal abnormalities are useful prognostic indicators.

63 The following are known predisposing factors in the development of leukaemia in humans:
   (a) Felty's syndrome.
   (b) Electromagnetism.
   (c) Viral infection.
   (d) Primary proliferative polycythaemia (polycythaemia rubra vera).
   (d) Exposure to benzene.

64 The following concern the presenting features of acute leukaemia — both acute myeloblastic leukaemia (AML) and acute lymphoblastic leukaemia (ALL):
   (a) The presenting symptoms are often due to bone marrow failure.
   (b) Fever can occur without obvious infection.
   (c) Enlargement of the spleen below the umbilicus is common.
   (d) Bone pain can be a feature.
   (e) Widespread lymphadenopathy is a diagnostic feature.

62 (a) **True**   Metaphase may be arrested by spindle poisons and the chromosomes can be stained by 'banding' techniques such as Giemsa (or G) banding.

(b) **True**   A long arm (q) and a short arm (p) are separated by a constriction known as the centromere.

(c) **False**   Translocations are reciprocal exchanges of genetic material between chromosomes resulting in shortening of one chromosome and lengthening of another. Chromosomal loss is referred to as deletion.

(d) **False**   Abnormalities may be random or clonal. Random changes describe different abnormalities in different cells. Clonal abnormalities are defined as the same abnormalities in different cells and indicate proliferation from a single cell (hence monoclonal as opposed to polyclonal).

(e) **True**   The type of abnormality helps to distinguish long-term survivors in certain types of leukaemia, for example acute lymphoblastic leukaemia (ALL) patients with high hyperdiploidy (> 50 chromosomes) have a better prognosis than those with hypodiploidy (< 46 chromosomes).

63 (a) **False**   Felty's syndrome is a combination of rheumatoid arthritis, splenomegaly and neutropenia.

(b) **False**   There is no evidence for a leukaemogenic effect of electromagnetism.

(c) **True**   Viral leukaemia is well-documented in avian and other mammalian species. In humans the strongest association between viral infection and leukaemia exists between HTLVI (human T lymphotopic virus type I) and T cell leukaemias. EBV and HTLVII are other viruses that may have an aetiological role in the development of leukaemia in humans.

(d) **True**   Acute myeloblastic leukaemia (AML) occurs as a terminal event in 10–15% of patients with primary polycythaemia.

(e) **True**   Benzene and its derivatives are potent bone marrow toxins producing aplasia and AML.

64 (a) **True**   The cardinal features are anaemia, bleeding due to thrombocytopenia and bacterial infection secondary to neutropenia.

(b) **True**   This may be due to an increased metabolic rate or the result of cytokines released from leukaemic or reactive cells. However, febrile neutropenic patients should be treated empirically with broad-spectrum antibiotics as many infective episodes in such patients are fatal if untreated.

(c) **False**   Only slight or occasionally moderate enlargement is present. It is more common in ALL (> 70%) than AML (50%).

(d) **True**   Due to bone marrow and periosteal infiltration. This is more common in children, who may also complain of joint pain. In these circumstances a misdiagnosis of juvenile rheumatoid arthritis or rheumatic fever may be made.

(e) **False**   Slight to moderate lymphadenopathy may be found in 80% of ALL patients but less than half of those with AML. The cervical nodes are most commonly affected and may be tender due to oropharangeal infection.

65 The following findings favour a diagnosis of AML rather than ALL:
   (a) A white cell count $> 100 \times 10^9/l$.
   (b) $> 30\%$ blasts in the bone marrow.
   (c) The presence of Auer rods.
   (d) Blast cells showing a positive cytochemical reaction using periodic acid Schiff (PAS).
   (e) The presence of cytoplasmic granulation in the abnormal cells.

66 In AML:
   (a) The absence of physical signs excludes the diagnosis of AML.
   (b) There are distinct morphological variants.
   (c) AML is less common in children than ALL.
   (d) Cytogenetic studies suggest the presence of clonal proliferation in many patients.
   (e) Some patients present with severe bleeding due to a major coagulopathy.

67 The following are statements about the treatment of AML:
   (a) Following chemotherapy 20% of patients are alive at 5 years.
   (b) Myelotoxicity is a major problem during treatment.
   (c) Elderly patients have the best prognosis.
   (d) Viral infections are common during treatment.
   (e) Meningeal relapse is common.

65 (a) **False** The presentation white cell count is very variable in both types of acute leukaemia and in either condition a white count $> 100 \times 10^9/l$ is a bad prognostic feature.

(b) **False** This is the level of blast cells in the bone marrow required to make a diagnosis of acute leukaemia. The diagnosis of AML or ALL depends on whether the blasts are myeloblasts or lymphoblasts.

(c) **True** Auer rods are rod-like structures with similar staining properties to primary granules with Romanovsky dyes and cytochemical stains. They are diagnostic of AML.

(d) **False** This property is a feature of ALL, in which cells have blocks of PAS- positive material in the cytoplasm. In contrast, AML blasts are positive with Sudan black and myeloperoxidase. These cytochemical tests are routinely employed to distinguish AML from ALL.

(e) **True** This indicates a degree of myeloid differentiation.

66 (a) **False** Some patients present with vague ill health and the diagnosis is subsequently established from examination of the peripheral blood and the bone marrow.

(b) **True** AML can be divided morphologically into several groups. The French–American–British (FAB) group currently recognise eight major variants (M0–M7) including erythroid and megakaryocytic varieties.

(c) **True** More than 80% of acute leukaemias in childhood are ALL.

(d) **True** Chromosomal abnormalities have been reported in at least 50% of patients with AML. Specialised techniques suggest that the true incidence of abnormalities is much higher. Some specific abnormalities have prognostic significance.

(e) **True** Disseminated intravascular coagulation (DIC) may occur in any infected patient with AML. Acute promyelocytic leukaemia (M3 AML by FAB classification) is characteristically associated with severe hypofibrinogenaemia and a major complex coagulopathy. This results in a higher early mortality in this particular type of AML.

67 (a) **True** 80% of patients achieve complete remission (CR) but the majority subsequently relapse, most within 2 years, only 20% of patients are alive at 5 years.

(b) **True** Most treatment schedules include several cytotoxic agents, the most constant of which are cytosine arabinoside and daunorubicin. The major problem with this combination of drugs is the depression of normal haemopoietic tissue whilst killing leukaemic cells.

(c) **False** Older patients are often unable to withstand the complications of intensive chemotherapy. In addition, daunorubicin — one of the most effective remission-inducing drugs — is cardiotoxic and can be dangerous in the elderly.

(d) **True** This is due to the immunosuppressive nature of the drugs. Herpes simplex virus infections occur in 30–40% of patients; they rarely become generalised or cause death but may cause fever and morbidity.

(e) **False** In contrast to ALL, meningeal relapse is found in only a minority of patients with AML and is usually limited to those patients presenting with a high white count ($> 100 \times 10^9/l$) and those cases with a monocytic component.

68 The following features are consistent with a diagnosis of ALL:
   (a) Blast cells in the cerebrospinal fluid.
   (b) Expression of B cell antigens by blast cells.
   (c) Evidence of a clonal T cell receptor gene rearrangement.
   (d) Hyperkalaemia.
   (e) A previous history of aplastic anaemia.

69 The following statements concern ALL:
   (a) The lymphoblasts in culture have a rapid cell cycle.
   (b) ALL occurs almost exclusively in children.
   (c) A mediastinal mass may be found.
   (d) Lymphoblasts are always found in the peripheral blood.
   (e) A high white cell count at presentation is a poor prognostic feature.

68 (a) **True**   Involvement of the CNS is present in 5% of patients at diagnosis and is an adverse prognostic feature.

(b) **True**   ALL may be of B or T lineage. The most common type of ALL (common ALL) has a pre-B phenotype, expressing early B cell antigens but not surface immunoglobulin. Common ALL accounts for more than 70% of both childhood and adult cases of ALL.

(c) **True**   During lymphoid development either immunoglobulin genes or T cell receptor genes rearrange during B or T cell development, respectively. Clonal rearrangements of these genes can be identified in DNA extracted from leukaemic cells, depending on whether the clone is of B or T cell origin. These rearrangements are usually absent in tumours of non-lymphoid origin, such as AML or carcinoma.

(d) **True**   This may occur in cases with a very high white cell count. Other features include hyperphosphataemia and hypocalcaemia.

(e) **True**   Some surviving patients with aplastic anaemia develop acute leukaemia, usually myeloblastic. However, at presentation a hypoplastic variant of ALL may mimic aplastic anaemia.

69 (a) **False**   DNA synthesis and cell replication is often much slower than for normal marrow cells. The increased tumour mass is due to lymphoblast accumulation, usually approaching 10^{11}–10^{12} cells by the time of diagnosis.

(b) **False**   There is a bimodal distribution with a peak in childhood and an increasing incidence in adults with advancing age, as for all other leukaemias.

(c) **True**   Most commonly in T cell ALL, in which the thymus may be very enlarged.

(d) **False**   Although careful examination of the blood film often reveals blast cells, they cannot be found in some cases. Bone marrow aspiration is therefore essential in all children presenting with the characteristic triad of anaemia, purpuric bleeding and infection.

(e) **True**   A high white cell count (particularly in excess of 20×10^{9}/l) with significant tissue infiltration reflects a higher leukaemic cell mass, which is associated with an increased incidence of early relapse.

70 The following concern the treatment of ALL:
  (a) It is possible to achieve a remission in 90% of children.
  (b) Maintenance therapy is unnecessary.
  (c) The prognosis in common ALL is worse than in B cell ALL.
  (d) Central nervous system relapse may occur during systemic remission.
  (e) Allogeneic bone marrow transplantation is the treatment of choice.

71 The following statements relate to infections in patients with haematological disorders:
  (a) Bacterial infections are uncommon during the remission induction phase of therapy of ALL.
  (b) Measles in children with ALL is a benign disorder.
  (c) *Pneumocystis carinii* is a common life-threatening infection in children with ALL.
  (d) Intravenous antibiotics should be administered to febrile neutropenic patients as soon as the results of bacterial cultures are available.
  (e) Prolonged periods of neutropenia in patients with AML are frequently associated with fungal infections.

72 The following are statements about the clinical findings in chronic myeloid leukaemia (CML):
  (a) Night sweats are common.
  (b) Splenomegaly is a major sign.
  (c) Patients commonly present with a thrombotic episode.
  (d) Bruising may occur despite a normal platelet count.
  (e) Lymphadenopathy is common at presentation.

70 (a) **True** Complete remission (CR) can be easily achieved without myelotoxicity in over 90% of cases using vincristine and prednisolone. The addition of further drugs such as daunorubicin produces even higher CR rates and may improve long-term survival.

(b) **False** The best results in childhood ALL have been obtained with continuous maintenance therapy for 2 to 3 years using methotrexate and 6-mercaptopurine.

(c) **False** This is the most common type of ALL in both children and adults and has the best prognosis. T cell ALL and null cell ALL may also be characterised by cell marker analysis (immunophenotyping).

(d) **True** Without prophylactic intrathecal methotrexate and cranial irradiation given to all patients early in the disease, 70–80% of children relapse. Despite this precaution up to 10% of children relapse in the CNS. The testes are another 'sanctuary' site where a relapse may occur.

(e) **False** The majority of patients with ALL are cured with conventional combination chemotherapy. Allogeneic transplantation from an HLA-matched sibling should be reserved for patients who relapse after standard treatment.

71 (a) **True** The cytotoxic regimens currently employed in ALL remission induction are less myelotoxic than those used for AML and produce less prolonged neutropenia. Thus, bacterial infection is uncommon during this phase of treatment in ALL, whilst it is common in AML.

(b) **False** This may be associated with severe complications, including pneumonitis and encephalitis. Children with ALL exposed to measles should be given high titre antimeasles globulin within 48 h of contact.

(c) **False** Until the introduction of prophylactic cotrimoxazole on three alternate days each week for the duration of treatment, infection with *Pneumocystis carinii* was a main cause of death in childhood ALL.

(d) **False** Sepsis in neutropenic patients may be rapidly fatal. Empirical treatment with broad-spectrum antibiotics should be instituted as soon as fever is documented. The results of cultures should not be awaited.

(e) **True** *Candida albicans* and aspergillosis are common but may be treated effectively with amphotericin.

72 (a) **True** These are due to the hypermetabolism associated with the vastly increased myeloid mass.

(b) **True** Moderate to marked enlargement is found in 85–90% of patients.

(c) **False** Hyperviscosity predisposing to thrombosis may be seen in patients with very high white cell counts (particularly > 500 × 10^9/l). This may present as venous thrombosis, priapism or stroke but such events are uncommon.

(d) **True** Platelet function may be impaired even if the count is normal or increased. In females, menorrhagia may be a presenting feature.

(e) **False** It may occur late in the disease.

73 The haematological findings in CML, at presentation, include:
   (a) A haemoglobin concentration often below 12 g/dl.
   (b) A white cell count usually > 100 × 10⁹/l.
   (c) Immature granulocytes found in the peripheral blood.
   (d) A high leucocyte (neutrophil) alkaline phosphatase (LAP).
   (e) An abnormal chromosome pattern, which is likely to be found in all haemopoietic cells.

74 The following features suggest a leukaemoid reaction rather than CML:
   (a) A predominance of myelocytes in the peripheral blood.
   (b) A basophil count of 3 × 10⁹/l.
   (c) The absence of a Philadelphia chromosome.
   (d) Toxic granulation.
   (e) A high LAP score.

75 The following relate to the clinical course and treatment of CML:
   (a) The average survival from the time of diagnosis is 3–4 years.
   (b) The clinical course is usually biphasic.
   (c) It is necessary for treatment to maintain the white cell count within normal limits.
   (d) Alpha interferon is the mainstay of treatment.
   (e) During transformation, the disease responds rapidly to treatment.

73 (a) **True**   Anaemia invariably develops. The haemoglobin concentration at presentation commonly lies between 8 and 10 g/dl.

(b) **True**   It is frequently in the range of 100–300 × 10⁹/l but may be higher.

(c) **True**   The white cell differential shows a full spectrum of myeloid cells ranging from blast cells, which may constitute up to 10% of the differential count, through promyelocytes, myelocytes, metamyelocytes and neutrophils. Eosinophilia, basophilia, thrombocytosis and nucleated red cells are also commonly found.

(d) **False**   The alkaline phosphatase activity normally found in neutrophils is virtually absent in CML. LAP is visualised cytochemically and scored according to the intensity of staining. The normal score lies between 20 and 100 but will vary from laboratory to laboratory.

(e) **True**   The Philadelphia chromosome (Ph′) is characteristically seen in cells of the granulocytic, monocytic, erythroid and megakaryocytic progenitors. Some lymphocytes also possess a Ph′ chromosome. This finding suggests that the leukaemic transformation arises in the pluripotent stem cell.

74 (a) **False**   A predominance of myelocytes as well as mature neutrophils is a feature of CML. Myelocytes are few in number in reactive leucocytosis.

(b) **False**   An absolute basophilic leucocytosis is frequently a feature of myeloproliferative disorders including CML.

(c) **True**   The Philadelphia chromosome is present in 95% of patients with CML.

(d) **True**   Primary granules are intensely stained.

(e) **True**   This is in keeping with toxic granulation and a reactive neutrophil leucocytosis.

75 (a) **True**   But may vary from a few months to 10 or more years.

(b) **True**   The initial chronic phase is followed by an accelerated phase with the development of fever, sweats, weight loss, bone pain and marrow failure.

(c) **False**   The aim of initial treatment is to reverse or prevent the onset of symptoms. There is no evidence that controlling the white cell count during the chronic phase prolongs survival.

(d) **False**   The value of interferon is as yet unproven. However, some patients become Philadelphia-negative but it is not yet known whether this will influence long-term survival.

(e) **False**   A feature of acceleration is resistance to treatment. However, 30% of patients developing very accelerated disease ('blast crisis') have a lymphoblast proliferation which in many instances will respond to ALL type therapy.

76 In a 52-year-old man with a monocyte count of $8.0 \times 10^9/l$, the following findings favour a diagnosis of chronic myelomonocytic leukaemia rather than a secondary monocytosis:
   (a) Generalised lymphadenopathy.
   (b) An increase in neutrophils.
   (c) Infection with tuberculosis.
   (d) Cytoplasmic vacuolation.
   (e) Thrombocytopenia.

77 The following relate to chronic lymphocytic leukaemia (CLL):
   (a) It is discovered as an incidental finding in many cases.
   (b) Hepatosplenomegaly may occur without lymph node enlargement.
   (c) Fever is a common presenting feature.
   (d) Haemolytic anaemia may complicate the disease.
   (e) Herpes zoster infections are quite common.

78 The following concern the pathological findings in CLL:
   (a) The white cell count is usually $> 100 \times 10^9/l$.
   (b) Mature lymphocytes infiltrate the bone marrow.
   (c) The lymphocytes have T cell characteristics.
   (d) 'Smear' cells in the peripheral blood are a typical finding.
   (e) A paraprotein is commonly detected.

79 The following relate to the course and treatment of CLL:
   (a) Treatment with chlorambucil is always indicated.
   (b) Most patients will live for 5 years.
   (c) The total body mass of leukaemic cells may be reduced by corticosteroid therapy.
   (d) The major risk is of developing a terminal blastic crisis.
   (e) Death is commonly due to infection.

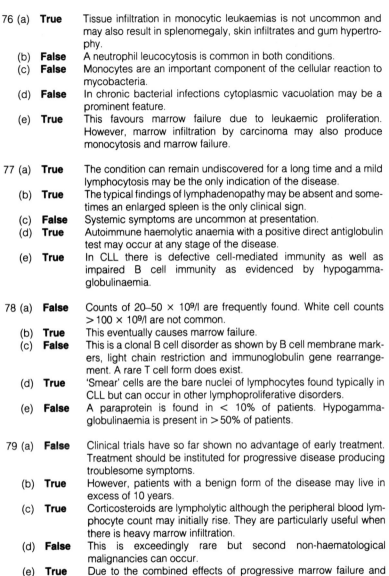

76 (a) **True**   Tissue infiltration in monocytic leukaemias is not uncommon and may also result in splenomegaly, skin infiltrates and gum hypertrophy.

  (b) **False**   A neutrophil leucocytosis is common in both conditions.

  (c) **False**   Monocytes are an important component of the cellular reaction to mycobacteria.

  (d) **False**   In chronic bacterial infections cytoplasmic vacuolation may be a prominent feature.

  (e) **True**   This favours marrow failure due to leukaemic proliferation. However, marrow infiltration by carcinoma may also produce monocytosis and marrow failure.

77 (a) **True**   The condition can remain undiscovered for a long time and a mild lymphocytosis may be the only indication of the disease.

  (b) **True**   The typical findings of lymphadenopathy may be absent and sometimes an enlarged spleen is the only clinical sign.

  (c) **False**   Systemic symptoms are uncommon at presentation.

  (d) **True**   Autoimmune haemolytic anaemia with a positive direct antiglobulin test may occur at any stage of the disease.

  (e) **True**   In CLL there is defective cell-mediated immunity as well as impaired B cell immunity as evidenced by hypogammaglobulinaemia.

78 (a) **False**   Counts of $20-50 \times 10^9/l$ are frequently found. White cell counts $>100 \times 10^9/l$ are not common.

  (b) **True**   This eventually causes marrow failure.

  (c) **False**   This is a clonal B cell disorder as shown by B cell membrane markers, light chain restriction and immunoglobulin gene rearrangement. A rare T cell form does exist.

  (d) **True**   'Smear' cells are the bare nuclei of lymphocytes found typically in CLL but can occur in other lymphoproliferative disorders.

  (e) **False**   A paraprotein is found in $<$ 10% of patients. Hypogammaglobulinaemia is present in $>$50% of patients.

79 (a) **False**   Clinical trials have so far shown no advantage of early treatment. Treatment should be instituted for progressive disease producing troublesome symptoms.

  (b) **True**   However, patients with a benign form of the disease may live in excess of 10 years.

  (c) **True**   Corticosteroids are lympholytic although the peripheral blood lymphocyte count may initially rise. They are particularly useful when there is heavy marrow infiltration.

  (d) **False**   This is exceedingly rare but second non-haematological malignancies can occur.

  (e) **True**   Due to the combined effects of progressive marrow failure and impaired humoral and cell mediated immunity. Chest and gut infections are both common.

80 The following are bad prognostic features in patients with CLL:
  (a) Bulky lymphadenopathy.
  (b) Autoimmune thrombocytopenia.
  (c) A lymphocyte count of 30×10^9/l.
  (d) Diffuse involvement of the bone marrow.
  (e) A family history of CLL.

81 Patients with myeloma frequently present with:
  (a) Painful bones.
  (b) Bleeding.
  (c) Infection.
  (d) Uraemia.
  (e) Peripheral neuropathy.

80 (a) **True**   This is indicative of disease at an advanced stage.

  (b) **False**   Thrombocytopenia due to marrow infiltration is a bad prognostic feature. However, thrombocytopenia secondary to hypersplenism or immune mechanisms does not in itself indicate a poor prognosis.

  (c) **False**   A lymphocyte count $< 50 \times 10^9/l$ suggests early disease. Subsequent follow-up to determine the lymphocyte doubling time will give further prognostic information. A doubling time in excess of 12 months is a relatively good prognostic marker.

  (d) **True**   Nodular and interstitial patterns of marrow involvement on histological sections may also occur and have a more favourable prognosis than diffuse involvement.

  (e) **False**   Of all the leukaemias, CLL has the highest familial incidence but this is of no prognostic significance.

81 (a) **True**   The disease is characterised by destruction of cortical and medullary bone. This causes bone pain and the typical 'punched out' osteolytic lesions. Diffuse osteoporosis may also occur. These changes can be associated with vertebral collapse and pathological fractures.

  (b) **False**   Bleeding is uncommon. When it occurs, it is usually due to abnormal platelet function due to 'coating' of the platelets by paraprotein or due to the latter interfering with the polymerisation of fibrin. Thrombocytopenia occurs late in the disease and is usually due to marrow infiltration or to treatment with cytotoxic drugs.

  (c) **True**   This is due to an immune paresis manifest as hypogammaglobulinaemia. Paraprotein 'coating' the neutrophils and impairing their function and marrow infiltration causing neutropenia are other reasons for infection.

  (d) **True**   One-quarter of patients presenting with myeloma are uraemic. More than 50% of patients with a serum creatinine concentration $> 200 \, \mu mol/l$ die within 3 months.

  (e) **False**   A painful sensory neuropathy may occur in a minority of patients. Other neurological manifestations may result from hyperviscosity or amyloid.

82 The following features are typically present in myeloma:
   (a) Rouleau formation in the blood film.
   (b) A plasma cell infiltrate of the bone marrow.
   (c) An IgA paraprotein.
   (d) Hypocalcaemia.
   (e) The serum alkaline phosphatase is usually raised.

83 The following statements relate to the treatment of myeloma:
   (a) All patients with a paraprotein require treatment.
   (b) Alkylating agents are effective cytotoxic agents in patients with myeloma.
   (c) It is not possible to alleviate the bone pain in myeloma.
   (d) Interferon therapy is curative in many patients.
   (e) Autologous bone marrow transplantation is often curative.

82 (a) **True**   This is very common and the blood film often has a blue background due to staining of the paraprotein fixed to the glass slide.

(b) **True**   More than 30% of the plasma cells in the bone marrow are commonly seen and, in conjunction with a paraprotein and lytic bone lesions, constitute the diagnostic triad for myeloma.

(c) **False**   Approximately 20% of patients present with an IgA and 55% with an IgG paraprotein. 20% secrete light chains only (Bence-Jones myeloma). Paraproteins of the other immunoglobulin classes are rare, as is non-secretory myeloma (i.e. no paraprotein or light chains in the urine). Patients with Bence-Jones only and non-secretory myelomas typically have a normal erythrocyte sedimentation rate (ESR) or plasma viscosity.

(d) **False**   Hypercalcaemia is common due to osteoclast-activating cytokines released from the plasma cells. Thus, presentation with anorexia, constipation, polyuria and dehydration is common. A high fluid throughput and corticosteroids are required urgently. Diphosphonates or calcitonin may be used.

(e) **False**   There is little osteoblastic activity associated with the bone disease. The normal serum alkaline phosphatase concentration is useful in distinguishing the hypercalcaemia of myeloma from that caused by hyperparathyroidism or metastatic carcinoma. However, the serum alkaline phosphatase will be raised in myeloma following a pathological fracture.

83 (a) **False**   Most patients with a solitary paraprotein do not have myeloma but simply a benign monoclonal gammopathy of uncertain significance. These patients do not require treatment but should be followed up because a minority will develop myeloma.

(b) **True**   Either melphalan or cyclophosphamide is highly effective at reducing the plasma cell mass. Successful treatment is usually accompanied by an improvement in symptoms, haematological findings and a fall in paraprotein concentration.

(c) **False**   Pain control is a major issue in the management of myeloma. In addition to opiates for analgesia, cytotoxic agents, corticosteroids, radiotherapy and non-steroidal anti-inflammatory agents may all be usefully employed to control bone pain.

(d) **False**   Few, if any, patients with myeloma are ever cured. The aim of therapy is to improve marrow function and prevent further tissue damage due to the tumour mass and paraprotein. Therapy is aimed at producing a stable 'plateau' phase. Recent studies indicate that interferon may usefully prolong the period of plateau phase and may be useful in conjunction with cytotoxic agents in achieving this plateau phase.

(e) **False**   Most patients with myeloma are elderly and any form of transplant procedure is inappropriate. Because it is not usually possible to completely eradicate disease from the marrow, autologous bone marrow transplant (BMT) (from self) is unlikely to be curative, although it may be used to prolong the plateau phase in young patients. Allogeneic transplantation (from donor) may offer a curative treatment for patients under the age of 45 years with a sibling donor and highly responsive disease.

84 In Waldenstrom's macroglobulinaemia (WM):
   (a) There is a polyclonal proliferation of B cells in the bone marrow.
   (b) Cerebral impairment is a characteristic feature.
   (c) Bence-Jones proteinuria occurs in more than 50% of patients.
   (d) Bleeding due to severe thrombocytopenia is common.
   (e) Early treatment with alkylating agents (e.g. chlorambucil, cyclo-
       phosphamide) is required.

85 The following are features of Hodgkin's disease:
   (a) The most common presentation is painless axillary lymphadenopathy.
   (b) Pruritus.
   (c) Basophilia
   (d) Lymphocytosis.
   (e) Bone marrow fibrosis.

86 In relation to Hodgkin's disease:
   (a) A diffuse infiltrate of large mononuclear cells is the typical histological
       appearance of involved lymph nodes.
   (b) Staging of the disease is mandatory.
   (c) Patients with fever and weight loss have disease very responsive to cytotoxic
       therapy and hence a better long-term prognosis.
   (d) Hodgkin's disease is incurable in 70% of patients.
   (e) Disease relapsing after many years is only curable by ablative cytotoxic
       therapy with bone marrow transplantation.

84 (a) **False** WM is a B-cell malignancy in which there is an accumulation of clonal lymphoplasmacytoid cells in the marrow and reticuloendothelial system.

(b) **True** Many patients present with features of hyperviscosity due to the accumulation of intravascular IgM paraprotein that is secreted by the clonal B cells. Impaired cerebral perfusion is rapidly corrected by removal of the paraprotein by plasmapheresis.

(c) **True** However, the quantity of light chain excreted is much less than in myeloma and renal impairment occurs in only 10% of patients.

(d) **False** Thrombocytopenia is a late manifestation but severe bleeding occurs early due to the paraprotein interfering with platelet adhesion and aggregation and fibrin polymerisation. In addition, hyperviscosity and cryoprecipitation lead to small vessel bleeding.

(e) **False** This is an insidious disease of the elderly. Viscosity should be controlled by judicious use of plasmapheresis and low-dose alkylating agents.

85 (a) **False** Painless cervical lymphadenopathy is present in 70% of patients. The axillary nodes are enlarged in 20% and inguinal nodes in 10%. It is worth noting that the nodes sometimes get smaller and then re-enlarge.

(b) **True** Hodgkin's disease may cause generalised pruritus.

(c) **False** Neutrophilia and eosinophilia are the typical white cell reactions seen.

(d) **False** Lymphopenia is found in 10–20% of cases and is an unfavourable prognostic indicator.

(e) **True** Bone marrow involvement with Hodgkin's disease is uncommon but when it occurs may be accompanied by an increase in reticulin fibres in the bone marrow.

86 (a) **False** Tumour histology is a disorganised mixture of lymphocytes, eosinophils, histiocytes and plasma cells interspersed with binucleate giant cells with large irregular nucleoli (Reed–Sternberg (RS) cells). When RS cells are surrounded by fibrous tissue they are described as lacunar cells, because of the appearance produced by shrinkage artefact.

(b) **True** The stage of the disease is the major prognostic factor and determines the initial treatment modality. Patients with stage I and limited stage II disease are best treated with radiotherapy whilst more advanced disease is best treated by combination cytotoxic chemotherapy (e.g. an alkylating agent in combination with procarbazine and corticosteroids). Staging laparotomy has now been superseded by imaging techniques such as computerised tomography.

(c) **False** These are 'B' symptoms and are an unfavourable prognostic feature. Patients with 'B' symptoms have disseminated disease and require combination cytotoxic chemotherapy.

(d) **False** Hodgkin's disease is curable in more than 70% of cases.

(e) **False** Disease relapsing after many years is usually responsive again to standard chemotherapy. High-dose therapy with bone marrow salvage is currently only being used for patients with resistant or rapidly relapsing disease.

87 The following relate to non-Hodgkin's lymphoma (NHL):
  (a) It is a tumour of T cells.
  (b) It rarely affects the bone marrow.
  (c) The stage of the disease is the most important prognostic factor.
  (d) The histological classification of NHL is simple.
  (e) Preservation of lymph node architecture is a major distinguishing feature from Hodgkin's disease.

88 In NHL:
  (a) Low-grade NHL requires intensive combination chemotherapy at an early stage.
  (b) High-grade NHL is best treated by radiotherapy.
  (c) Prophylactic treatment to the CNS is not required.
  (d) Fever and weight loss are uncommon in high-grade NHL.
  (e) 70% of patients with low-grade lymphoma are curable.

89 Toxic effects of radiation therapy include the following:
  (a) Nausea.
  (b) Pneumonitis.
  (c) Intellectual impairment.
  (d) Hyperthyroidism.
  (e) The development of acute myeloblastic leukaemia.

87 (a) **False** NHL may result from a malignant proliferation of any constituent cell of lymphoid tissue. This includes B cells, T cells and histiocytes. B cell lymphomas are by far the most common.

(b) **False** In contrast to Hodgkin's disease. The bone marrow is frequently involved because NHL is often at an advanced stage at the time of diagnosis.

(c) **False** Stage is important but the histological grade is the most important prognostic factor.

(d) **False** NHL may be classified morphologically or immunologically. Most classification symptoms are complex and varied but some degree of unification of systems has been attempted with the introduction of the Working Formulation. In this international system NHL is graded as low, intermediate or high. This system has prognostic significance and determines treatment modality.

(e) **False** Whilst nodal architecture is preserved in some lymphomas (follicular), in the majority nodal architecture is disrupted. In general, tumour growth correlates with architectural disruption and hence diffuse lymphomas have a worse prognosis than follicular lymphomas.

88 (a) **False** Low-grade lymphomas have an insidious onset and are slowly progressive. Treatment is only required when there are symptoms or impaired organ function.

(b) **False** High-grade lymphomas are usually treated with intensive combination cytotoxic chemotherapy. Using regimens such as CHOP (cyclophosphamide, hydroxydaunorubicin, Oncovin, prednisolone) 60–70% of patients achieve complete remission and 30% require no further treatment.

(c) **False** High-grade lymphomas may relapse in or involve the CNS. Certain histological types are particularly likely to relapse in the CNS and in these cases prophylactic treatment to the CNS is indicated.

(d) **False** These are common features in high-grade NHL and indicate advanced aggressive disease.

(e) **False** Few if any patients with low-grade NHL are cured. However, treatment may not be required initially and these lymphomas can often be controlled for many years with low-dose, single-agent chemotherapy (e.g. chlorambucil).

89 (a) **True** Nausea, vomiting and diarrhoea are early effects and potent antiemetic and antidiarrhoeal drugs should be administered prophylactically.

(b) **True** This is a serious late effect. Lung shielding can be used to reduce the dose to the lungs.

(c) **True** This may occur in children, for example those with ALL receiving prophylactic cranial irradiation.

(d) **False** Hypothyroidism and other endocrine failures may occur.

(e) **True** There is an increased incidence of AML several years after radiotherapy. This is seen particularly in those patients who also received alkylating agents for ovarian carcinoma, myeloma and Hodgkin's disease. Environmental exposure to irradiation is also leukaemogenic.

90 The following concern acquired aplastic (hypoplastic) anaemia:
   (a) There is commonly a pancytopenia.
   (b) A bone marrow aspirate can appear to be of normal cellularity.
   (c) Splenomegaly is a consistent feature at the time of diagnosis.
   (d) The reticulocyte count is usually $> 80 \times 10^9/l$ (normal range 30–100 $\times$ $10^9/l$).
   (e) Ferrokinetic studies are required for diagnosis.

91 The following are statements about aplastic (hypoplastic) anaemia:
   (a) The cause is usually due to drug treatment.
   (b) About 40–50% of the patients die within 6 months.
   (c) Immunosuppressive therapy increases the risk of infection and is contraindicated.
   (d) Bone marrow transplantation (BMT) should be performed as soon as possible following a diagnosis of aplastic anaemia.
   (e) Blood products are of minimal value in the management of aplastic anaemia.

92 The following results were found on examining the blood of a 46-year-old woman: Hb 8.5 g/dl, MCV 90 fl, MCH 29 pg, WBC 2.1 $\times$ $10^9/l$, platelets 90 $\times$ $10^9/l$. The spleen was not palpable. The following conditions are likely to give this picture:
   (a) Aplastic (hypoplastic) anaemia.
   (b) Hypersplenism.
   (c) Untreated primary myelofibrosis.
   (d) Megaloblastic anaemia.
   (e) Systemic lupus erytheomatosus.

90 (a) **True**   This is the classic blood picture but often one cell line is more severely reduced than the others.

(b) **True**   A hypocellular marrow is typical but active areas may occur. A trephine biopsy is necessary to assess cellularity accurately.

(c) **False**   The presence of splenomegaly should always raise doubts about the diagnosis of aplastic anaemia.

(d) **False**   Reticulocytes are almost absent from the peripheral blood.

(e) **False**   Ferrokinetic studies using Fe59 show delayed plasma clearance and reduced marrow utilisation but are not required for diagnosis.

91 (a) **False**   Only 50% are due to drugs, chemicals, irradiation or viral infection.

(b) **True**   Only 25–30% of patients have a partial remission but may relapse; complete remission is less frequent.

(c) **False**   50% of patients with aplastic anaemia have a useful remission following therapy with antilymphocyte globulin. The addition of cyclosporin or anabolic steroids may improve the results. This finding suggests an immune basis for many cases of aplastic anaemia.

(d) **False**   Immunosuppressive therapy is the treatment of choice in patients with less severe forms of aplastic anaemia. The clearest indication for allogeneic BMT is the young patient with severe aplastic anaemia particularly with neutrophils $< 0.2 \times 10^9/l$. For these patients BMT offers a better long-term survival than immunosuppressive therapy.

(e) **False**   Prolonged survival depends upon transfusion of blood components when they are clinically indicated. Leucodepleting filters should be used with red cell and platelet transfusions as exposure to white blood cells is responsible for HLA alloimmunisation and consequently refractoriness to platelet transfusions and an increased risk of graft failure should allogeneic BMT be performed.

92 (a) **True**   Pancytopenia with a normochromic, normocytic anaemia without splenomegaly may be due to aplastic anaemia although a slight macrocytosis may be present.

(b) **False**   The spleen is usually enlarged and palpable, although there is no correlation between the size of the spleen and the degree of hypersplenism and hence pancytopenia.

(c) **False**   One would expect to find significant splenomegaly. Other forms of marrow infiltration commonly produce pancytopenia without splenomegaly, e.g. acute leukaemias, lymphoma, myeloma and secondary carcinoma.

(d) **False**   Pancytopenia can be a presenting feature but there should be a red cell macrocytosis.

(e) **True**   Pancytopenia may result from immune destruction of cells or myelofibrosis. Hypersplenism may also result when splenomegaly occurs.

93 The following concern patients with persistently high haemoglobin concentrations (i.e. > 18 g/dl in males and > 16.5 g/dl in females):
  (a) The red cell mass/plasma volume should always be determined.
  (b) The total blood volume is usually increased in primary proliferative polycythaemia.
  (c) Blood viscosity remains unaltered in primary polycythaemia.
  (d) Platelet function in primary polycythaemia is usually normal.
  (e) The high haemoglobin could be due to an abnormality of the oxygen affinity of haemoglobin.

94 The following are important features concerning the diagnosis of primary proliferative polycythaemia (PPP) (polycythaemia rubra vera):
  (a) The white cell count is usually > 30 × 10^9/l.
  (b) Haematuria is a constant finding.
  (c) Splenomegaly is found in 70% of patients.
  (d) The arterial oxygen saturation is > 90%.
  (e) The following results are consistent with the diagnosis of primary polycythaemia: Hb 14 g/dl, packed cell volume (PCV) 0.50, MCV 72 fl, MCH 20 pg, red blood cell (RBC) 7.01 × 10^{12}/l, neutrophils 12.5 × 10^9/l, platelets 470 × 10^9/l.

93 (a) **True** It is essential to determine whether there is a relative or absolute polycythaemia. In the former the high haemoglobin is due to a reduction in the plasma volume — found in dehydration, following long-term diuretic treatment and in polycythaemia of stress. In true polycythaemia the red cell mass is increased. This may result from erythropoietin drive (e.g. hypoxia, Epo-secreting tumour) or autonomous production by the marrow (primary proliferative polycythaemia, also known as polycythaemia rubra vera).

(b) **True** The total blood volume is composed of the plasma volume and red cell mass. The latter is usually > 30% of the predicted value. The plasma volume can be normal or increased. This accounts for many of the clinical features, including the red face, conjunctival suffusion and the engorged veins seen on fundoscopy.

(c) **False** Viscosity increases with increasing haematocrit. It is this increase that is partly responsible for the high incidence of thrombosis that characterises the disease.

(d) **False** More than half the patients have abnormal platelet function as judged by platelet aggregation studies. In many patients aggregation is decreased but in others it is increased. The latter, together with the classically increased platelet count, also predisposes to thrombosis.

(e) **True** One of the most common causes of a mild erythrocytosis (i.e. increase in red cells unaccompanied by neutrophilia or thrombocytosis) is the presence of carboxyhaemoglobin in tobacco smokers. There are also rare familial haemoglobinopathies characterised by increased oxygen affinity which are compensated for by an increased red cell mass (e.g. Hb Chesapeake).

94 (a) **False** It is uncommon for the white cell count to be as high as this but in 60% of patients it is 10–25 × 10⁹/l. Primary polycythaemia is a myeloproliferative disorder characterised by a stem cell abnormality that subsequently involves erythroid, myeloid and megakaryocyte cell lines but with the predominant feature of the disease being an increased red cell mass.

(b) **False** The urine should be examined in all patients with polycythaemia. Haematuria may be due to a renal carcinoma or polycystic kidney disease, both of which can be associated with increased erythropoietin levels and secondary polycythaemia with a raised red cell mass.

(c) **True** The presence of splenomegaly is a major feature and helps distinguish primary polycythaemia from other secondary and relative polycythaemias.

(d) **True** This is in contrast to the low oxygen saturation often found in chronic pulmonary disease or cyanotic congenital heart disease, both of which produce a secondary polycythaemia with a raised red cell mass.

(e) **True** The neutrophil leucocytosis and the relatively high haemoglobin with iron-deficient indices are suggestive of iron deficiency in a patient with primary polycythaemia.

95 The following concern the management of PPP:
   (a) The prognosis without treatment is good.
   (b) Venesection has an important role.
   (c) Pruritus can be difficult to treat.
   (d) Young patients should be treated with radioactive phosphorus.
   (e) Chronic myeloid leukaemia (CML) occurs as a terminal event in 10% of patients.

96 The following statements relate to primary myelofibrosis:
   (a) Reticulin fibres are increased in the bone marrow.
   (b) The development of myelofibrosis can be preceded by primary polycythaemia.
   (c) Extramedullary haemopoiesis is a cardinal feature of the disease.
   (d) The disease is often found incidentally.
   (e) Palpable splenomegaly is usual.

95 (a) **False**   The average survival without treatment is 18 months. Death is usually due to thrombotic disease or haemorrhage.

(b) **True**   Venesection is a rapid method of reducing viscosity. A unit of blood (500 ml) can be taken daily for 2 days and subsequently every alternate day until the packed cell volume is brought down < 0.50. It may be necessary to give a plasma expander at the same time as the venesection to prevent hypotension (isovolaemic venesection).

(c) **True**   This is a common and distressing symptom. It may be related to histamine metabolism. Aspirin, H_2-receptor antagonists, ultraviolet light and interferon have been used to treat the pruritus.

(d) **False** ^{32}P is leukaemogenic and should only be used in elderly patients who cannot attend hospital regularly for other forms of treatment.

(e) **False**   CML following primary polycythaemia is uncommon, but acute myeloblastic leukaemia occurs in about 10% of patients as a terminal event. The high incidence of acute leukaemia has been attributed to the mutagenic effects of ^{32}P and alkylating agents. Antimetabolites and enzyme inhibitors such as hydroxyurea may be useful and are not leukaemogenic.

96 (a) **True**   The normal fine reticulin pattern is lost and replaced by coarse bands of fibres. Myelofibrosis may also occur in carcinoma, secondary to tuberculosis and following exposure to benzene (secondary myelofibrosis).

(b) **True**   10–20% of patients with primary polycythaemia subsequently develop myelofibrosis. Some patients can present with features of both disorders.

(c) **True**   It occurs in the liver and spleen but may be present in other tissues.

(d) **False**   The patient usually has symptoms attributable to splenomegaly and frequently they have constitutional symptoms especially weight loss and night sweats.

(e) **True**   The spleen is usually easily felt and in many patients may be massive. It is extremely uncommon for the spleen to be impalpable but when this is the case, imaging techniques usually show splenic enlargement.

97 In relation to myelodysplastic syndromes:
    (a) There is often a neutrophil leucocytosis.
    (b) Vitamin B_{12} levels are often low.
    (c) Transformation to AML is common.
    (d) Exposure to carcinogens is common.
    (e) The percentage of blasts in the bone marrow is often increased.

98 In the myelodysplastic syndromes:
    (a) Blood product support is of minimal value.
    (b) Infection only occurs in neutropenic patients.
    (c) Median survival is 10–20 years.
    (d) Ring sideroblasts in the bone marrow are a bad prognostic factor.
    (e) There may be a marked monocytosis.

99 The following changes are visible in the peripheral blood film following splenectomy:
    (a) Target cells.
    (b) Howell–Jolly bodies.
    (c) Thrombocytopenia.
    (d) Lymphocytosis.
    (e) Red cells containing haemosiderin.

97 (a) **False** The myelodysplastic syndromes are a group of related disorders in which there is dysplastic maturation of one or more cell lines. Haemopoiesis is ineffective and whilst the bone marrow is usually hypercellular there is peripheral blood cytopenia.

(b) **False** Haematinic deficiency must be excluded before diagnosing a myelodysplastic syndrome. Dysplastic features in the presence of low vitamin B_{12} or folate levels would suggest megaloblastosis.

(c) **True** The myelodysplastic syndromes are due to clonal repopulation of the bone marrow and clonal evolution to overt acute myeloblastic leukaemia is not infrequent. For this reason this group of disorders is also referred to as 'preleukaemia' or 'smouldering leukaemia'.

(d) **False** The majority of patients have no identifiable exposure to carcinogens. However, exposure to alkylating agents, irradiation and organic solvents is associated with the development of myelodysplasia.

(e) **True** The percentage of blasts is one of the criteria by which the myelodysplastic syndromes may be classified. By definition the percentage of blasts is < 30% as a value greater than this is arbitrarily defined as acute leukaemia.

98 (a) **False** Red cell and platelet transfusions are the mainstay of treatment in the symptomatic patient. There is as yet no definitive treatment for advancing disease, although strategies ranging from ablative cytotoxic chemotherapy to experimental differentiation therapy are being evaluated.

(b) **False** Infections are common due to neutrophil dysfunction. Similarly, platelet dysfunction may result in bleeding.

(c) **False** Survival is very variable ranging from a median of 6 months for patients with > 20% blasts to 6 years with < 5% blasts in the marrow.

(d) **False** The longest survival is in patients with few blast cells and large numbers of ringed sideroblasts, so called refractory anaemia with ringed sideroblasts or primary acquired sideroblastic anaemia.

(e) **True** Myelodysplasia may be associated with a proliferative monocytosis in which the peripheral blood monocyte count exceeds $1.0 \times 10^9/l$. The condition is then termed chronic myelomonocytic leukaemia.

99 (a) **True** After splenectomy many red cells gain membrane lipid and consequently surface area and in dried blood films this leads to 'target cell' formation. An assortment of other red cell morphological abnormalities occurs.

(b) **True** Howell–Jolly bodies are nuclear remnants that are present in approximately 1% of red cells following splenectomy and other hyposplenic states.

(c) **False** The platelet count rises rapidly after splenectomy reaching a peak between 1 and 2 weeks. Within a few weeks the platelet count returns to high normal levels in the majority of individuals.

(d) **True** Following splenectomy there is a neutrophilia in the first week but subsequently the leucocytosis is mainly due to increased lymphocytes, monocytes and eosinophils.

(e) **True** 'Pappenheimer' bodies consisting of ferritin are present in small numbers of red cells following splenectomy.

100 The following statements relate to hypersplenism:
(a) Neutropenia is uncommon.
(b) Palpable splenomegaly is invariably present.
(c) The bone marrow is hypocellular.
(d) The plasma volume is reduced.
(e) The blood count usually returns to normal after splenectomy.

101 The peripheral blood film may show features of hyposplenism in:
(a) Inflammatory bowel disease.
(b) Rheumatoid arthritis.
(c) Premature infants.
(d) Newly diagnosed hereditary spherocytosis.
(e) Sickle-cell disease.

102 The following factors reduce thrombus formation:
(a) Thromboxane A2.
(b) Plasmin.
(c) Antithrombin III.
(d) Circulatory stasis.
(e) Decreased concentrations of coagulation factors.

100 (a) **False** In hypersplenism, splenic enlargement is accompanied by one or more cytopenias. Whilst each cell line may be affected to a variable degree, pancytopenia is common.

(b) **False** Although unusual, the absence of a palpable spleen does not exclude hypersplenism.

(c) **False** The marrow is hyper- or occasionally normocellular, reflecting increased haemopoiesis.

(d) **False** An expansion of the plasma volume accompanies splenic enlargement and may contribute to the development of cytopenia.

(e) **True** Correction of cytopenia by splenectomy is a characteristic of hypersplenism, although recovery may be partially delayed due to the gradual reduction in plasma volume.

101 (a) **True** Although it is more commonly found in gluten-induced enteropathy (coeliac disease).

(b) **False** Splenic enlargement with hypersplenism is well-recognised in seropositive rheumatoid disease.

(c) **True** Splenic function is not optimal until the second month of life. This results in an increased susceptibility to bacterial infections in the newborn, particularly in premature infants.

(d) **False** Hereditary spherocytosis (HS) is a red cell membrane disorder in which a defect of the cytoskeleton results in a progressive loss of membrane lipid. These cells are 'lysed' in the spleen and splenic hyperplasia may occur.

(e) **True** Hyposplenism occurs in children with sickle-cell anaemia due to repeated infarction of the spleen (autosplenectomy).

102 (a) **False** Thromboxane A2 is a prostaglandin metabolite produced by platelets with potent vasoconstrictor and platelet aggregatory activity. Aspirin may exert its antithrombotic effect by inhibiting thromboxane generation.

(b) **True** Plasmin is the effector molecule of the fibrinolytic system. A deficiency of plasminogen, the precursor of plasmin, appears to be associated with a tendency to thrombosis.

(c) **True** Antithrombin III is one of the body's natural anticoagulants. It neutralises activated coagulation enzymes, especially thrombin and factor Xa. It is a member of the SERPIN group of molecules (serine protease inhibitors).

(d) **False** Stasis potentiates thrombosis, e.g. postoperatively, cardiac failure.

(e) **True** Warfarin exerts its antithrombotic effect by reducing functional levels of the vitamin K-dependent coagulation factors.

103 The following factors are thought to potentiate thrombus formation:
     (a) Prostacyclin (PGI$_2$).
     (b) Thrombocythaemia.
     (c) Damaged vascular endothelium.
     (d) Depressed reticuloendothelial function.
     (e) Inhibitors of fibrinolysis.

104 The following concern abnormal bleeding due to thrombocytopenia:
     (a) Cutaneous bleeding is typical.
     (b) Bleeding from a superficial skin cut is often prolonged.
     (c) Gastrointestinal haemorrhage is uncommon.
     (d) Bleeding following tooth extraction is delayed.
     (e) A history of drug ingestion is important.

103 (a) **False**   PGI$_2$ is a major prostaglandin synthesised by endothelial cells. It is a powerful vasodilator and inhibits platelet adhesion and aggregation.

   (b) **True**   Patients with persistently high platelet counts, particularly when due to myeloproliferative disorders, have an increased risk of thromboembolism.

   (c) **True**   The 'anticoagulant' properties of the endothelium are lost and the thrombogenic subendothelium is exposed. Normal endothelium inhibits thrombus formation by concentrating natural anticoagulants such as antithrombin III and activated protein C, on the endothelial surface, secreting prostacyclin and releasing activators of the fibrinolytic system.

   (d) **True**   Patients with disseminated intravascular coagulation have a depressed reticuloendothelial clearance system. It is thought that failure of the system to remove activated clotting factors further aggravates thrombus formation, whilst failure to remove fibrin degradation products interferes with polymerisation of fibrin and consequently bleeding is more pronounced.

   (e) **True**   A decreased fibrinolytic potential is generally thought to be a risk factor for the development of thromboembolism. Families with recurrent venous thrombosis and high plasminogen activator inhibitor (PAI) levels have been reported.

104 (a) **True**   Spontaneous pin-point petechial haemorrhages (purpura) or multiple small bruises are common in the presence of severe thrombocytopenia ($< 30 \times 10^9$/l).

   (b) **True**   This is particularly common. The bleeding time is the time taken for bleeding to cease after a standardised skin incision and is prolonged in both thrombocytopenia and qualitative platelet defects. It may also be prolonged in vascular defects.

   (c) **False**   Bleeding from mucous membranes is common, leading to frequent gingival bleeding and epistaxis. Occasionally, haematemesis or malaena may occur but in such cases additional gastrointestinal pathology should be considered.

   (d) **False**   Bleeding is usually immediate. Bleeding due to coagulation factor deficiency is often delayed and more persistent than thrombocytopenic bleeding.

   (e) **True**   As well as causing thrombocytopenia, e.g. thiazides, quinine, drugs that inhibit platelet function, e.g. aspirin, non-steroidal anti-inflammatory drugs, may exacerbate bleeding due to thrombocytopenia.

105 Neonatal thrombocytopenia is associated with:
   (a) Intrauterine infection.
   (b) Maternal immune thrombocytopenic purpura.
   (c) Skeletal abnormalities in the infant.
   (d) Sickle-cell disease.
   (e) Maternal alloantibodies to platelet-specific antigens.

106 The following are general statements concerning platelets:
   (a) Of the platelets produced by the bone marrow at any one time 30% are pooled within the spleen.
   (b) The normal platelet life-span is about 120 days.
   (c) Platelet concentrates can be used to control thrombocytopenic bleeding for up to 4 weeks after donation.
   (d) Patients commonly become refractory to repeated platelet transfusions.
   (e) Impaired platelet function following aspirin is irreversible.

105 (a) **True**   Thrombocytopenia may be associated with other features of congenital infection – TORCH syndrome (toxoplasma, rubella, cytomegalovirus, herpes simplex).

   (b) **True**   Immune destruction of maternal platelets by IgG antibodies may also result in transplacental transfer of antibody and destruction of fetal platelets.

   (c) **True**   Congenital megakaryocytic hypoplasia may be associated with skeletal and other congenital malformations.

   (d) **False**   Sickle-cell disease is not associated with thrombocytopenia. Sickle-cell disease is not manifest at birth as beta globin chain synthesis is not predominant until 4–6 months later.

   (e) **True**   Analogous to the maternal red cell antibody production responsible for haemolytic disease of the newborn, transplacental passage of fetal platelets may occasionally result in maternal alloimmunisation to platelet antigens and consequently destruction of fetal platelets by maternal antibodies. This condition is known as neonatal alloimmune thrombocytopenia (NAIT) and is most frequently caused by antibodies to the PIA_1 antigen.

106 (a) **True**   Due to their small size, platelets take a circuitous route through the red pulp and splenic cords of the spleen — a much slower pathway than the direct route through the splenic sinusoids. The net result is a considerable splenic pool of platelets, which may be expanded if there is significant splenomegaly.

   (b) **False**   The normal platelet life-span is about 10 days.

   (c) **False**   Platelets may be obtained from one donor by cell separation techniques or by pooling platelet concentrates from four or five blood donors. These platelets are useful in arresting thrombocytopenic bleeding, if correctly stored for up to 5 days.

   (d) **True**   Refractoriness to platelet transfusions may occur for a variety of reasons, including fever, sepsis, hypersplenism, consumption and after repeated administration the development of human leucocyte antigen (HLA) alloantibodies. Leucodepletion of red cell and platelet products may reduce the incidence of human leucocyte antigens (HLA)-alloimmunisation as platelets themselves only weakly express HLA-antigens.

   (e) **True**   Aspirin irreversibly acetylates cyclo-oxygenase and inhibits prostaglandin metabolism. Platelets are unable to synthesise cyclo-oxygenase and, once exposed to aspirin, lose aggregatory activity for the remainder of their life-span.

107 The following are causes of thrombocytopenic purpura:
   (a) Henoch–Schoenlein purpura.
   (b) Aplastic (hypoplastic) anaemia.
   (c) Systemic lupus erythematosus (SLE).
   (d) Malaria.
   (e) Haemorrhagic disease of the newborn.

108 The following are causes of non-thrombocytopenic bleeding:
   (a) Congenital platelet storage pool disorders.
   (b) Scurvy.
   (c) Serum sickness.
   (d) Hereditary haemorrhagic telangiectasia.
   (e) Folate deficiency.

107 (a) **False** This condition is thought to be an allergic response to a preceding infection. There is widespread evidence of a vasculitis resulting in a raised purpuric-like rash appearing on the extensor surfaces of the limbs accompanied by polyarthritis, abdominal pain, bloody diarrhoea and haematuria. The platelet count is normal.

   (b) **True** Thrombocytopenia can occur in any disease where there is a reduction in the number of megakaryocytes in the marrow. This may be due to idiopathic aplastic anaemia, the effect of drugs, chemicals and ionising radiation or due to marrow infiltration (e.g. in leukaemia, lymphoma, myelomatosis or secondary carcinoma).

   (c) **True** Thrombocytopenia may result from antiplatelet antibody production, the interaction of immune complexes with the platelet membrane, hypersplenism or inadequate marrow production.

   (d) **True** Due to consumption of platelets. A degree of thrombocytopenia is extremely common but most severe in falciparum infection.

   (e) **False** This is due to a deficiency of the vitamin K-dependent coagulation factors. Approximately one-third of healthy full-term infants are vitamin K deficient and, without vitamin K administration, two-thirds have become deficient by day 4. The platelet count is normal.

108 (a) **True** Platelet numbers in these disorders are normal but platelet function is defective due to a deficiency of platelet stored substances required for normal platelet secretion and aggregation. Spontaneous bleeding is uncommon but prolonged bleeding after surgery is usual.

   (b) **True** Bleeding is usually the presenting feature due to defective collagen synthesis in the vessel wall. A perifollicular petechial distribution is typical.

   (c) **True** Fever, arthralgia, lymphadenopathy, urticaria and purpura occur after exposure to heterologous proteins or drugs. Purpura results from vasculitis.

   (d) **True** In this autosomal dominant condition the development of small thin walled angiomatous malformations in the skin, mucous membranes and organs leads to chronic blood loss from the gastrointestinal tract. The lesions can be distinguished from purpura as they blanch on pressure.

   (e) **False** Folate deficiency results in ineffective megaloblastic haemopoiesis with resulting thrombocytopenia.

109 The following are true of the haemolytic uraemic syndrome (HUS):
    (a) Intravascular haemolysis occurs.
    (b) Many cases in children result from toxin-producing bacterial infection.
    (c) Disseminated intravascular coagulation is invariably present.
    (d) Administration of fresh frozen plasma is indicated.
    (e) Most affected children require long-term dialysis for chronic renal failure.

110 The following characterise bleeding due to haemophilia A (factor VIII:C deficiency):
    (a) Epistaxis.
    (b) Haemarthrosis.
    (c) Muscle haematomas.
    (d) Delayed bleeding after trauma.
    (e) A family history of bleeding.

109 (a) **True** There is severe red cell fragmentation associated with haemoglobinaemia, methaemalbuminaemia, haemoglobinuria and absent haptoglobin.

(b) **True** The so-called 'classic' form follows a prodromal phase of bloody diarrhoea resulting from infection with 'verotoxin' producing *Escherichia coli* 0157. HUS may also occur following other bacterial and viral infections.

(c) **False** Microvascular platelet thrombi occur predominantly in the kidney in the absence of coagulation factor consumption. This phenomenon is unexplained.

(d) **True** Management of renal failure, hypertension and anaemia is required. In some cases administration of plasma or indeed plasma exchange improves both the renal and haematological manifestations. Presumably a toxic agent is removed or a missing factor is restored.

(e) **False** Despite the severity of the acute illness, most affected children recover completely.

110 (a) **False** Spontaneous bleeding into mucous membranes is uncommon in coagulation factor deficiencies.

(b) **True** Haemarthrosis into hinge joints is characteristic of severe coagulation factor deficiencies. The knee is the most common site, except in children under the age of 2 years, where the ankle is most frequently affected.

(c) **True** These are often apparently spontaneous, although the trauma that precipitated them may have passed unnoticed by the patient.

(d) **True** Haemostasis may be achieved initially only to be followed by rebleeding when the platelet plug, which is poorly reinforced with fibrin, is disrupted

(e) **True** A family history is present in the majority of patients with congenital haemophilia, however new mutations are common.

111 The following concern haemophilia A (factor VIII deficiency):
   (a) If a male haemophiliac marries a normal female all their daughters will be carriers.
   (b) The severity of bleeding is related to the factor VIII concentration.
   (c) Chronic arthritis is uncommon.
   (d) Neuropathy is a recognised complication.
   (e) It occurs more commonly than Christmas disease.

112 The following are features of haemophilia A:
   (a) Von Willebrand protein cannot be detected in the blood.
   (b) Carriers have normal levels of factor VIII coagulant activity.
   (c) Antibodies to factor VIII occur in 5–10% of patients.
   (d) Abnormal liver function tests are present in at least 30% of adults.
   (e) Aspirin is a useful drug for controlling the pain associated with acute haemarthrosis.

111 (a) **True** As it is a sex-linked disease, the male must pass his affected X chromosome to his daughters.

(b) **True** Severe haemophilia occurs only in those with factor VIII concentrations < 1 u/dl. Spontaneous haemorrhage becomes increasingly uncommon as the factor VIII level approaches 5 u/dl. Above this concentration most haemorrhages are related to trauma or surgery.

(c) **False** Chronic haemophilic arthropathy often follows repeated bleeding into the knees and ankles. This complication can be minimised by prompt treatment as soon as the haemorrhage commences. The major advantage of 'home' therapy is that the haemophiliac administers their own factor VIII replacement, which they keep at home or at work, as soon as bleeding occurs.

(d) True Bleeding into the soft tissues can involve nerves. Common sites are the forearm, resulting in a radial nerve lesion and the thigh, involving the femoral nerve. Evidence of damage to vital anatomical structures should be considered whenever a haemophiliac has a soft tissue haemorrhage. This is particularly important if the haematomas involves the head or neck.

(e) **True** Severe haemophilia occurs in 1:25 000 of the population, although milder forms are more common. The ratio of haemophilia to Christmas disease (factor IX deficiency) is about 5:1, which reflects the size of the respective genes.

112 (a) **False** The factor VIII molecule consists of two components: the factor VIII coagulant protein (VIII:C) and the large multimeric von Willebrand factor (vWF). The von Willebrand protein is necessary for platelet adhesion to subendothelial structures and also protects the coagulant protein from proteolysis in the circulation. Thus VIII:C levels are reduced in both haemophilia A (VIII:C gene defect) and von Willebrand disease (vWF gene defect), whilst the vWF level is reduced only in von Willebrand disease.

(b) **False** The average VIII:C level in female carriers is 50% of normal. However, there is considerable overlap with the normal range. A carrier state may be suggested by high vWF level compared to VIII:C level in a female with a family history of haemophilia A. The most reliable method of detecting the carrier state is by tracking the haemophilia gene through the family using probes on DNA digests that give a particular pattern for the haemophilia haplotype in each family (RFLP – restriction fragment length polymorphism).

(c) **True** Antibodies ('inhibitors') to factor VIII render standard replacement therapy ineffective. The management of such patients is extremely difficult and the development of inhibitors is associated with a high morbidity and mortality.

(d) **True** The majority of haemophiliacs have been infected with hepatitis viruses through the use of blood products. The number of patients with chronic active hepatitis who develop cirrhosis remains to be seen.

(e) **False** The platelet inhibitory effect of aspirin increases the bleeding tendency. Haemophiliacs should not take aspirin-containing compounds.

113 Patients with severe haemophilia, FVIII:C < 1 u/dl (normal >50 u/dl):
   (a) Should be advised not to ride a bicycle because of the risk of injury.
   (b) Should have an urgent CT scan of the head as a first priority if they develop severe headache.
   (c) Should be given prophylactic treatment if bleeds occur frequently in a joint.
   (d) May develop haematuria.
   (e) Should not be immunised because intramuscular injections cause severe muscle haematomas.

114 The following are true of von Willebrand disease:
   (a) It is inherited as a sex-linked disorder.
   (b) The bleeding time may be normal.
   (c) Platelet aggregation in response to adenosine diphosphate (ADP) is typically reduced.
   (d) Cryoprecipitate is the treatment of choice for a bleeding episode.
   (e) Intrapartum haemorrhage is often problematic.

113 (a) **False**   Many severe haemophiliacs benefit from the exercise of non-contact sports. Activities that may result in intracranial haemorrhage or haemarthrosis are contraindicated: rugby, boxing, wrestling.

    (b) **False**   If there is suspicion of intracranial bleeding factor VIII replacement therapy should be administered as the first priority. Intracranial haemorrhage is a major cause of death in severe haemophilia.

    (c) **True**   Prophylactic therapy may reduce the frequency of bleeding and permit 'healing' of a 'target joint'.

    (d) **True**   Two-thirds of severe haemophiliacs have at least one episode of haematuria. Treatment in the first instance is an increased fluid intake for several days to reduce the risk of urinary clot formation and obstruction. Investigation is not indicated unless haematuria is chronic or recurrent.

    (e) **False**   Intramuscular injections are generally avoided but immunisation by the subcutaneous route is safe. All patients should be immunised against hepatitis B.

114 (a) **False**   The von Willebrand factor (vWF) gene is on chromosome 12 and von Willebrand disease is inherited in an autosomal dominant pattern. Heterozygotes have vWF levels of approximately 50% of normal with a mild to moderate bleeding disorder. Homozygotes have levels < 5% and a severe bleeding disorder.

    (b) **True**   Whilst a long bleeding time may result from deficient von Willebrand protein and suboptimal platelet–subendothelial adhesion, a bleeding time at the limit of normal is not uncommon.

    (c) **False**   Platelet aggregation in response to agonists is normal whilst platelet agglutination in response to ristocetin is defective. Ristocetin facilitates binding of plasma vWF to the vWF receptors on the platelet surface. By virtue of its large size and multiple binding sites, vWF forms a bridge between platelets and agglutinates them.

    (d) **False**   Cryoprecipitate is a rich source of vWF but carries the risk of transmission of infectious diseases. Desmopressin (DDAVP) and antifibrinolytic agents are used to treat mild von Willebrand disease, thus avoiding the use of blood products, whilst virus inactivated factor VIII concentrates are reserved for patients with severe disease.

    (e) **False**   vWF levels rise throughout pregnancy and the majority of females with von Willebrand disease have normal levels by the time of delivery.

115 These coagulation results were obtained from a 26-year-old male patient: prothrombin time 13 s (control 12 s), partial thromboplastin time 60 s (control 40 s). These results suggest the following diagnosis:
   (a) Factor VII deficiency.
   (b) Factor XI deficiency.
   (c) Factor XII deficiency.
   (d) Factor IX deficiency.
   (e) Severe liver disease.

116 The following coagulation results were obtained from a 50-year-old woman: prothrombin time 45 s (control 12 s), partial thromboplastin time 63 s (control 41 s). The possible causes are:
   (a) Factor V deficiency.
   (b) Established oral anticoagulant therapy.
   (c) Prolonged obstructive jaundice.
   (d) Lack of factor X.
   (e) Massive blood transfusion.

117 The following results were obtained from a 50-year-old man who had no previous history of abnormal or excessive bleeding: prothrombin time > 90 s (control 12 s), partial thromboplastin time > 90 s (control 40 s), thrombin time > 90 sec (control 11 s). The most likely diagnoses are:
   (a) Congenital afibrinogenaemia.
   (b) Heparin excess.
   (c) A 'clot' in the sample.
   (d) Warfarin overdose.
   (e) Disseminated intravascular coagulation (DIC).

115 (a) **False**   Fibrin formation in plasma may be initiated by the addition of thromboplastin or exposure to a foreign surface. Addition of thromboplastin quickly leads to fibrin formation (prothrombin time – PT) and is dependent on factor VII and independent of the contact factors and factors VIII and IX (the so-called extrinsic pathway). Exposure to a foreign surface leads to a slower generation of fibrin (the partial thromboplastin time – PTT) and is dependent on the presence of all the factors in the coagulation cascade with the exception of factor VII (the so-called intrinsic system). Therefore a long PTT does not result from a deficiency of factor VII.

   (b) **True**   A long PTT will result from a significant deficiency of any of the contact factors (XI, XII, prekallikrein).

   (c) **True**   See answer (b).

   (d) **True**   This degree of prolongation would suggest moderate, rather than severe, factor IX deficiency.

   (e) **False**   Liver disease results in a complex disturbance of haemostasis, which includes multiple coagulation factor deficiencies. A prolongation of the prothrombin time due to low levels of factor VII generally precedes prolongation of the partial thromboplastin time.

116 (a) **True**   Factor V is a cofactor in the generation of thrombin by activated factor X. Its position in the final common pathway will result in prolongation of both PT and PTT in deficiency states.

   (b) **True**   The vitamin K-dependent factors II, VII, IX and X will all be reduced.

   (c) **True**   Again, the vitamin K-dependent factors will be reduced due to poor absorption of vitamin K, which is fat soluble.

   (d) **True**   See answer (a).

   (e) **True**   Due to dilution. Both factors V and VIII are absent in stored blood.

117 (a) **False**   The addition of thrombin to plasma converts fibrinogen to fibrin and the time taken for clot formation to occur is a measure of both the fibrinogen level and the rate of conversion to fibrin (thrombin time). Although the results of the laboratory tests in this case would be found in congenital afibrinogenaemia the absence of any previous bleeding excludes the diagnosis.

   (b) **True**   The thrombin time and partial thromboplastin time are sensitive to the effects of heparin. In the presence of heparin excess the prothrombin time is also prolonged.

   (c) **True**   Clot formation results in depletion of fibrinogen. The resulting serum is incapable of clotting.

   (d) **False**   Severe warfarin overdose may prolong the PT and PTT to such a degree but fibrinogen levels are not reduced and fibrin formation is normal. Thus the thrombin time is always normal.

   (e) **True**   These results would indicate a most severe consumptive coagulopathy. Severe thrombocytopenia and elevated levels of fibrin degradation products would also be found.

118 The following are statements concerning disseminated intravascular coagulation (DIC):
   (a) Thrombosis is rare.
   (b) Bleeding can be a major feature.
   (c) Fragmentation of red cells may be observed on a blood film.
   (d) A normal platelet count excludes DIC.
   (e) Treatment with heparin is usually indicated.

119 The following concern chronic autoimmune thrombocytopenic purpura (AITP):
   (a) Patients may be asymptomatic.
   (b) Intracerebral haemorrhage is common.
   (c) Moderate splenomegaly is usual.
   (d) Menorrhagia is rare.
   (e) It often follows an upper respiratory tract infection.

118 (a) **False** The condition is characterised by initiation of coagulation resulting in widespread fibrin deposition in the microcirculation. Large vessel thrombosis may also occur.

(b) **True** Intravascular coagulation consumes coagulation factors resulting in bleeding. The precise clinical picture will depend upon the nature of the provoking factors and the degree of compensatory fibrinolysis, e.g. acute bleeding can occur in pregnancy where sudden release of amniotic fluid or placental thromboplastin into the circulation causes rapid consumption of fibrinogen and platelets. In contrast, deep vein thrombosis is common in patients with carcinoma. A mixed picture of thrombosis and bleeding can be seen in DIC associated with septicaemia, especially that caused by *Neisseria meningitidis*.

(c) **True** The mechanism of fragmentation has not been defined. Shortened red cell survival may lead to anaemia (microangiopathic haemolysis).

(d) **False** Almost any combination of coagulation abnormalities can occur in partially compensated DIC. It is important to perform a full assessment of coagulation, including fibrin degradation products.

(e) **False** The underlying cause should be treated. Coagulation replacement therapy may reduce bleeding.

119 (a) **True** Since the inclusion of a platelet count in the automated full blood count, AITP is often picked up incidentally in adults and is chronic and asymptomatic.

(b) **False** Intracerebral haemorrhage is rare, occurring in well under 1% of cases.

(c) **False** Splenomegaly is rarely found.

(d) **False** Menorrhagia is a common feature of thrombocytopenia and may be the presenting complaint.

(e) **False** This is particularly common in children but there is rarely a history of infection in adults. Acute autoimmune thrombocytopenic purpura in children with a history of 'viral' illness is often termed postinfectious thrombocytopenia and the spontaneous remission rate of 90% contrasts with the 10% rate seen in adult chronic AITP.

120 The following are true of the management of AITP:
  (a) The patient's current medication is not relevant.
  (b) Other than a full blood count, detection of platelet-bound antibody (IgG and IgM) is the only peripheral blood test required.
  (c) A bone marrow aspirate is a necessary investigation.
  (d) Megakaryocyte numbers are reduced in the bone marrow.
  (e) Splenectomy is the initial treatment of choice.

121 The following changes in coagulation take place during a normal pregnancy:
  (a) Fibrinolysis is increased.
  (b) Plasma fibrinogen is decreased.
  (c) Factor VIII:C is increased.
  (d) Antithrombin III concentration is normally increased.
  (e) Fibrin is deposited in the walls of the spiral arteries.

120 (a) **False**   Several drug induced thrombocytopenias have an immune mechanism, notably that associated with thiazide diuretics and quinine.

(b) **False**   It is particularly important to detect diseases that may be associated with AITP in adults, such as systemic lupus, HIV infection and lymphoma and to refute other mechanisms of thrombocytopenia, such as B_{12} or folate deficiency, liver disease or low grade consumptive coagulopathy.

(c) **False**   If the haemoglobin and white cell count are normal and presentation is typical, many clinicians do not perform a marrow examination in children.

(d) **False**   Megakaryocyte numbers are increased to compensate for the increased peripheral destruction.

(e) **False**   First-line treatment is prednisolone, initially 1 mg/kg body weight, slowly reducing after 2 weeks. Some patients remit permanently after this. Splenectomy is most useful in steroid-responsive cases that relapse but should be avoided in children under the age of 6 years. High-dose intravenous immunoglobulin is useful in haemorrhagic steroid refractory cases and preoperatively but the remission is usually short lived (3–4 weeks).

121 (a) **False**   Fibrinolytic activity is decreased in early pregnancy remaining low throughout with a rapid return to normal postdelivery.

(b) **False**   Fibrinogen production doubles during pregnancy if due allowance is made for the increase in plasma volume.

(c) **True**   Of the coagulation factors VIII:C shows the greatest increase but significantly elevated concentrations of factor VII and X are also noted.

(d) **False**   Most of the inhibitors of coagulation are little affected by pregnancy. The net result of all these changes is a hypercoagulable state. In consequence, thrombosis is a major cause of maternal death.

(e) **True**   Fibrin deposits replace the normal elements of the vessel wall. This facilitates expansion of the vessels to accommodate increasing placental blood flow during pregnancy. The presence of fibrin is probably an important factor in arresting blood flow at placental separation.

122 Patients on warfarin:
    (a) Would be advised not to get pregnant.
    (b) Should limit their alcohol intake.
    (c) Require an assessment of anticoagulant control once a week.
    (d) Should have their dose increased when co-trimoxazole is prescribed.
    (e) Should stop warfarin 1 week before surgery.

123 A 75-year-old man with a Bjork–Shiley mitral valve replacement has been well-controlled on warfarin. He presents before his next appointment with epistaxis and is found to have an international normalised ratio (INR) > 8.0.
    (a) His correct INR should be 3.0–4.5.
    (b) He should be questioned regarding the colour of the tablets he is taking.
    (c) He should be given factor VIII concentrate immediately.
    (d) He should be given 10 mg of intravenous vitamin K.
    (c) His warfarin should be stopped and his INR repeated after 1 week.

122 (a) **True** However, for women on life-long warfarin who wish to have children, a pregnancy test should be performed if they miss a period and, if pregnant, subcutaneous heparin should be substituted for warfarin.

(b) **True** Whilst alcohol excess may inhibit liver enzymes and potentiate the warfarin effect, a moderate consumption of alcohol has no effect.

(c) **False** Once stabilised, monitoring of anticoagulation can be safely performed once every 6–12 weeks. The degree of anticoagulation is determined by the international normalised ratio (INR), which is a measurement based on the prothrombin time.

(d) **False** Many drugs either inhibit or potentiate the effect of warfarin and anticipation of dose alteration and careful monitoring of warfarin are required with changes of medication. Co-trimoxazole inhibits the metabolism of warfarin, thus potentiating the anticoagulant effect. A dose reduction is usually required.

(e) **False** Depending on the type of surgery it is often possible to reduce the degree of anticoagulation to achieve an INR of 2.0 and perform operative procedures without an excessive degree of haemorrhage.

123 (a) **True** It is recommended that patients with mechanical (metal) heart valves in the mitral position have a target INR of between 3.0–4.5.

(b) **True** Elderly patients may have impaired vision or become confused. Discrepancies between what the doctor thinks the patient is taking and what the patient is actually taking are common, even in previously well-controlled patients.

(c) **False** Warfarin interferes with the action of factors II, VII and IX and X (the vitamin K-dependent factors).

(d) **False** This dose of vitamin K would completely reverse the warfarin effect in 12–18 h, leaving the patient at risk from valve thromboemboli. If the epistaxis is severe, 1 mg of intravenous vitamin K should be administered and the INR repeated in 24 h. For immediate reversal, administration of fresh frozen plasma is required.

(e) **False** The patient may become unanticoagulated and thus be at risk of valve thromboembolism. If the warfarin is stopped the INR should be checked regularly and warfarin reintroduced to maintain anticoagulation.

124 In relation to thromboembolic disease:
   (a) A patient developing a spontaneous pulmonary embolus (PE) requires life-long anticoagulation.
   (b) A 45-year-old patient undergoing surgery with a deep vein thrombosis (DVT) 15 years earlier is at low risk of further thrombosis.
   (c) A patient found to have protein C deficiency during a family study requires life-long anticoagulation.
   (d) A patient with a previous DVT who is no longer taking warfarin develops a second DVT. They should be anticoagulated to achieve an INR of 3.0–4.5.
   (e) The maximum risk period for thrombosis in a pregnant woman is the first trimester.

125 The following are true of heparin:
   (a) The usual method of controlling intravenous administration is measurement of the partial thromboplastin time.
   (b) It is essential to monitor prophylactic subcutaneous heparin.
   (c) Osteoporosis is rarely seen after heparin administration.
   (d) Thrombocytopenia may occur after administration of small doses.
   (e) Protamine sulphate can be used to reverse the heparin effect.

126 The following are true of DDAVP (desmopressin):
   (a) Given intravenously it shortens the bleeding time in most patients with von Willebrand disease.
   (b) It increases the FVIII:C level in patients with severe haemophilia.
   (c) Given intravenously it increases fibrinolysis.
   (d) It can be used to shorten the bleeding time in patients with uraemia.
   (e) It can be used repeatedly in patients with haemophilia A undergoing surgery.

124 (a) **False**   For a single episode of thromboembolic disease patients require a finite period of anticoagulation. Patients usually receive anticoagulants for 6–12 months after a PE.

(b) **False**   Patients over the age of 40 with a history of thromboembolic disease are at high risk of thrombosis during and following surgery.

(c) **False**   Deficiency of natural anticoagulants increases the risk of thromboembolic disease. However, a number of people with deficiencies suffer no thrombotic event and therefore anticoagulation should not be instituted in the absence of thromboembolic disease.

(d) **False**   Standard anticoagulation to achieve an INR of 2.0–3.0 is required. It is only necessary to increase the intensity of anticoagulation if a patient develops a thromboembolic event whilst on anticoagulants.

(e) **False**   The maximum risk period is at the end of the pregnancy and particularly in the first few weeks following delivery.

125 (a) **True**   Heparin binds and greatly increases the 'natural' anticoagulant effect of antithrombin III, leading to neutralisation of activated coagulation factors. There is a dose-dependent prolongation of the partial thromboplastin time in response to heparin.

(b) **False**   It is not usual to monitor low-dose prophylactic subcutaneous heparin but therapeutic doses of heparin may be administered subcutaneously and require careful monitoring.

(c) **True**   Osteoporosis occasionally appears to be related to prolonged administration of heparin (in excess of 15 000 units a day for more than 5 months). The mechanism is unknown.

(d) **True**   Even heparinising an intravenous line can cause mild thrombocytopenia in a sensitised patient. Heparin-induced thrombocytopenia is moderate and immune-mediated. A rarer form due to platelet activation by heparin is severe and associated with arterial and venous thrombosis.

(e) **True**   Such reversal is rarely necessary as heparin is a heterogeneous mixture of polysaccharides with biological half-lives varying between 30 and 120 min. It is rarely necessary to do more than temporarily stop a heparin infusion to reduce anticoagulation.

126 (a) **True**   This is due to a release of vW multimers from the endothelium. However, it is ineffective in severe von Willebrand disease when there are no stored multimers.

(b) **False**   By functional assay there is no increase in FVIII:C levels as there is too little normal factor VIII available. It does, however, increase FVIII:C levels two-to four-fold in mild haemophiliacs (FVIII:C > 5 iu/dl) by a mechanism that is unclear.

(c) **True**   This is due to the release of plasminogen activator from the endothelium. The effect is short-lived however (< 10 min) and does not counteract the haemostatic effect of DDAVP. This response can be used to assess endothelial-mediated fibrinolytic activity in patients with recurrent thromboembolic disease.

(d) **True**   von Willebrand protein levels are already normal or increased in uraemia and therefore the mechanism of action of DDAVP is unexplained.

(e) **False**   Tachyphylaxis occurs, i.e. a reduction in response with repeated doses.

127 Tranexamic acid, an antifibrinolytic agent, is useful in the following situations:
   (a) To cover dental extractions in patients with a bleeding tendency.
   (b) To control menorrhagia/epistaxis in patients on warfarin.
   (c) Gastrointestinal haemorrhage in a patient with no known coagulation defect.
   (d) Haematuria in thrombocytopenia or coagulation factor deficiency.
   (e) Haemarthrosis or intracranial haemorrhage in haemophiliacs.

128 High-dose intravenous immunoglobulin is routinely indicated for:
   (a) A patient with a platelet count of $45 \times 10^9/l$ due to chronic autoimmune thrombocytopenia.
   (b) Prolonged thrombocytopenia after cytotoxic therapy.
   (c) Someone who has suffered a needle-stick injury from a hepatitis B surface-antigen-positive person.
   (d) Hypogammglobulinaemia.
   (e) Asymptomatic patients infected with human immunodeficiency virus (HIV).

129 Requirements for blood donors in the UK are:
   (a) The haemoglobin concentration should be > 14 g/dl,
   (b) The donor should not have been abroad during the previous 6 months.
   (c) The donor should not have been pregnant within the previous year.
   (d) The donor should never have been jaundiced.
   (e) The donor should have no haemoglobinopathy trait.

127 (a) **True**   It is usually started immediately prior to extraction and continued for 5–7 days afterwards. It is important to prevent secondary haemorrhage due to infections as well.

(b) **False**   Tranexamic acid should not be given to patients on warfarin as it is potentially prothrombotic. It is contraindicated in patients with thromboembolic disease, including coronary artery disease.

(c) **True**   Tranexamic acid has been shown to reduce blood loss and red cell transfusion requirements in patients with active peptic ulcers.

(d) **False**   It may cause ureteric obstruction and clot colic.

(e) **False**   These patients require coagulation factor replacement. Tranexamic acid may be useful in these patients for mild external 'surface' bleeding.

128 (a) **False**   High-dose immunoglobulin therapy will elevate the platelet count in > 80% of patients with autoimmune thrombocytopenia but the median duration of action is short, with a peak platelet count at 12 days. Such therapy may be useful for treating bleeding episodes or preparing patients for surgery.

(b) **False**   Immunoglobulin does not affect thrombocytopenia resulting from inadequate marrow production.

(c) **False**   Specific high titre antihepatitis B immunoglobulin is given to non-immune individuals.

(d) **True**   Immunoglobulin replacement therapy prevents recurrent infection.

(e) **False**   These patients have high immunoglobulin levels but poor specific antibody responses to infection and may be functionally hypogammaglobulinaemic. The role of immunoglobulin therapy has not yet been clarified. It may, of course, be used to treat associated immune thrombocytopenia or neutropenia.

129 (a) **False**   The accepted levels are 13.5 g/dl in males and 12.5 g/dl in females.

(b) **False**   Donors who have been to certain tropical areas where there is a high incidence of infectious diseases that can be transmitted by blood products are asked to defer their donation until 6 months after their return. Travel to most countries is not a contraindication to donation.

(c) **True**   This is to prevent excessive demands on the volunteer's iron stores.

(d) **False**   Donors with a history of jaundice or hepatitis occurring more than 1 year previously may be accepted if hepatitis B surface antigen is not detectable in the blood by the most sensitive techniques available.

(e) **False**   Donors with haemoglobinopathy traits are not excluded unless anaemic. Certain antigens, and also antibodies, are more common in some ethnic populations and it is highly desirable to have donations from ethnic groups with a high incidence of thalassaemias or haemoglobinopathies that require transfusion support.

130 Blood donations in the UK are tested for antibodies to:
  (a) HIV.
  (b) HTLVI.
  (c) Hepatitis C.
  (d) Syphilis.
  (e) Malaria.

130 (a) **True**   However, donor self-exclusion is of major importance in reducing the risk of transfusion-related transmission of HIV.

(b) **False**   Routine testing for HTLVI is not performed in the UK. Like HIV this is a lymphocytotrophic virus and antibodies present in the serum infer donor infection. Infection is common in Afro-Caribbean and Japanese individuals and is associated with the development of adult T cell lymphoma/leukaemia in some carriers, and spastic paraparesis.

(c) **True**   However, the majority of transfusion associated hepatitis is now due to hepatitis C (non-A non-B hepatitis). The introduction of testing for exposure to hepatitis C will hopefully reduce the incidence of this complication.

(d) **True**   The risk of developing syphilis following transfusion of blood from a donor with active syphilis is small, as spirochetes do not survive more than four days at 4°C. However, evidence of exposure to syphilis is a 'surrogate' marker of exposure to HIV.

(e) **False**   Antibodies to malaria antigens are not routinely measured. Prevention of transfusion-associated malaria is mainly by donor exclusion within 6 months of travelling to an endemic area. Individuals born or brought-up in endemic areas are excluded for 3 years after arrival in the UK and are tested for antibody in some transfusion centres.

131 The following are general statements about transfusion and blood groups:
   (a) Donor blood is usually collected into heparin, which acts an an anticoagulant.
   (b) Most fatal ABO incompatible blood transfusions are the result of rare subgroups giving rise to serological errors.
   (c) Anti-A and anti-B are usually absent from the serum of group O neonates.
   (d) The following blood groups (ABO, Rh(D) and MN) are from a mother, child and putative father: mother A Rh(D) positive MN; child O Rh(D) negative NN; putative father A Rh(D) positive NN. The results exclude paternity.
   (e) After blood has been stored for 5 weeks, at least 70% of transfused red cells should be retained in the circulation 24 h after transfusion.

131 (a) **False**   Heparin is inactivated during the first 24 h following donation so that the blood clots in the bag. Donor blood is collected into citrate–phosphate dextrose (CPD) solution. If blood is collected in a triple pack system, the plasma can be separated into an empty pack and an optimal additive solution added to the red cells from the third pack, e.g. saline adenine glucose manitol (SAG-M), which improves the viability and flow properties of the plasma reduced red cells.

(b) **False**   Most result from administrative errors either due to sample misidentification prior to ABO typing and cross-matching or product/patient misidentification prior to transfusion. All samples should be carefully labelled with several points of identification and prior to transfusion the group and compatibility label on the red cell transfusion pack should be compared with the documented ABO type of the patient. The patient identification details on the issue card accompanying the blood product should be compared with the patient's notes and identification wristband.

(c) **True**   The strength of anti-A and anti-B gradually increases from birth to adult levels over the first 5 years. The stimulus is thought to be the presence of antigens in the environment, which are similar to blood group substances. The antibodies develop when the corresponding A or B antigen is absent. These antibodies are said to be 'naturally occurring', in contrast to those produced after exposure to heterologous red cells (e.g. transfusion or in pregnancy, when they are termed 'immune').

(d) **False**   These blood groups are inherited in a simple mendelian fashion. Both mother and putative father could have the ABO genotype of AO and could have a child with blood group O. Similarly, a person inherits two Rhesus haplotypes from each parent. The two most common are CDe and cde. By current English transfusion nomenclature Rhesus positivity relates solely to the presence of the D antigen. A Rhesus-positive father and mother could each be heterozygous for the D antigen and could therefore produce a Rhesus-negative child. Similarly, the child in this case has inherited an N antigen from each parent. The case of paternity is therefore not disproved. The rules that apply in excluding paternity are: (i) a man is excluded if both he and the mother lack an antigen that is present in the child; (ii) a man is excluded if antigens that he must pass to his offspring are not present in the child. DNA 'fingerprinting' has now largely replaced red cell phenotyping for paternity testing.

(e) **True**   This is the internationally recognised minimum criterion for adequate storage of red cell products.

132 The following concern basic immunological reactions in blood group serology:
  (a) Anti-A agglutinates group A erythrocytes when they are suspended in saline.
  (b) Low ionic strength solutions (LISS) are widely used to speed up cross-match procedures.
  (c) The antiglobulin (Coombs') test detects antibodies on the red cell membrane that fail to agglutinate the red cells when they are suspended in saline.
  (d) The direct antiglobulin test identifies *in vivo* sensitisation of red cells.
  (e) The indirect antiglobulin test is used in the standard cross-match procedure.

133 The following statements concern reactions occurring during a blood transfusion:
  (a) Complement-mediated red cell lysis accompanies the administration of ABO-incompatible blood.
  (b) Renal failure may follow the transfusion of ABO incompatible blood.
  (c) An isolated febrile reaction, occurring 30 min after commencing a transfusion, is usually due to Rhesus incompatibility.
  (d) Sudden extreme hypotension may indicate that the transfused blood is contaminated with bacteria.
  (e) Anaphylaxis may result from blood transfusion.

132 (a) **True**   When washed and resuspended in saline, red cells are negatively charged and surrounded by a 'cation cloud', leading to repulsion. By virtue of its large size, naturally occurring IgM antibody can span the gap between the red cells.

    (b) **True**   LISS reduces the density of the cation cloud surrounding red cells suspended in saline, allowing greater sensitisation by positively charged antibody. The cross-match time has been reduced from between 60 and 90 min to 10–15 min. LISS also enhances certain weak antigen–antibody reactions.

    (c) **True**   IgG antibody will not agglutinate red cells suspended in saline. In the Coombs' test anti-human globulin (AHG) is added to the antibody-sensitized cells. This recognises and binds to IgG acting as a 'linchpin' between antibody on the surface of the adjacent red cells and allowing agglutination to take place.

    (d) **True**   The red cells are washed in saline and AHG added. Agglutination indicates a positive direct Coombs' test and sensitisation of red cells *in vivo*.

    (e) **True**   The indirect Coombs' test. Donor red cells are incubated *in vitro* with the recipient's serum to ascertain whether the latter contains IgG antibodies that could prematurely destroy the donor cells if they were transfused. After incubation the donor cells are washed and AHG is added. If agglutination is present then the donor red cells are incompatible with the recipient and should not be transfused.

133 (a) **True**   Anti-A and anti-B are IgM antibodies that activate complement. This causes red cell lysis with haemoglobinaemia and haemoglobinuria. Vasoactive peptides are liberated as complement is activated, resulting in flushing of the face, headache, dyspnoea, constricting pain in the chest, lumbar pain and hyperperistalsis.

    (b) **True**   Renal failure may result from an ABO incompatible blood transfusion. The damage to the kidneys may result from the hypotensive effects of vasoactive peptides, complement depletion or glomerular obstruction by red cell stroma. Hypotension must be corrected and urine output maintained.

    (c) **False**   This type of reaction is probably due to proteins other than red cell antigens. In some patients the symptoms can be minimised by paracetamol. Leucocyte antibodies may cause recurrent febrile transfusion reactions. In such cases leucodepleted blood products should be administered.

    (d) **True**   This fortunately rare occurrence is usually due to contamination of a unit of blood with Gram-negative bacilli capable of proliferating at 4°C.

    (e) **True**   Whilst urticaria is one of the most common immunological complications of blood transfusion, anaphylaxis is rare. This is usually due to the reaction between normal IgA in the donor plasma and class specific anti-IgA antibody in the plasma of an IgA deficient recipient. The incidence of the latter in the normal population is 1:1000.

134 The following are complications of rapid massive blood transfusion:
   (a) Electrocardiographic abnormalities.
   (b) Metabolic acidosis.
   (c) Abnormal bleeding.
   (d) Hypothermia.
   (e) A significant alteration in haemoglobin function.

135 The following are statements about blood and blood products:
   (a) Whole blood transfusion is essential when treating massive haemorrhage.
   (b) Plasma-reduced blood (packed cells) has an inferior post-transfusion survival compared with whole blood.
   (c) Cryoprecipitate contains fibrinogen.
   (d) Blood product replacement therapy in patients with disseminated intravascular coagulation (DIC) is contraindicated.
   (e) Fresh donor blood may be used for sick neonates within 1 h of collection from previously screened donors.

134 (a) **True**   The combination of hypocalcaemia, hyperkalaemia and hypothermia can result in electrocardiographic changes and, in extreme cases, cardiac arrest.

(b) **False**   Despite the low pH of stored blood, acidosis in the recipient is rare because metabolism of citrate produces alkalosis. Acidosis is more likely to result from circulatory failure. Potential problems exist at very high transfusion rates (10 u/h) in patients who are shocked.

(c) **True**   This is usually due to dilution of coagulation factors and platelets. If a transfusion is likely to continue beyond 8–10 units, consideration should be given to replacement therapy with fresh frozen plasma and platelet concentrates. The requirement for such therapy depends on the rate of transfusion and therefore coagulation tests and platelet counts should be measured to determine the need for replacement therapy.

(d) **True**   The transfusion of cold blood in large quantities can lower the body 'core' temperature. This can be avoided by the use of a blood warmer.

(e) **False**   2,3-diphosphoglycerate (2,3-DPG) is the major determinant of oxygen unloading by haemoglobin. The problem of low levels of 2,3-DPG in stored blood has largely been eliminated by the addition of adenine together with saline and manitol (SAG-M), in which the cells are suspended following the removal of the plasma for component therapy. Near normal levels of 2,3-DPG are now maintained for most of the shelf-life of red cells.

135 (a) **False**   Concentrated red cells may be used to correct anaemia. Volume expansion may be achieved with crystalloid or colloid solutions. Haemostasis may be supported by administration of platelet concentrates and fresh frozen plasma. Certain coagulation factors and platelets are not functional in stored whole blood. Giving packed cells, platelet concentrates and fresh frozen plasma (component therapy) is more beneficial than whole blood.

(b) **False**   The survival of red cell concentrates is identical to that of whole blood. Red cell concentrates are indicated for the correction of anaemia.

(c) **True**   In addition to factor VIII, factor XIII and fibronectin. Virus-inactivated fibrinogen concentrate will soon supersede the use of cyroprecipitate for fibrinogen replacement therapy.

(d) **False**   Component therapy will replace deficient factors and may reduce bleeding. There is a theoretical risk that replacement therapy will increase thrombosis.

(e) **False**   It is unacceptable to use fresh blood that has not been tested for transfusion transmitted infections. Component therapy is possible even in the smallest infant. Transfusion centres produce 'baby packs' to minimise waste.

136 The following statements relate to blood products:
  (a) 20% albumin solution is useful in the treatment of nephrotic syndrome.
  (b) Specific immunoglobulins prepared from donor plasma in the convalescent phase of infectious disease can be used to confer active immunity.
  (c) The administration of 4.5% albumin solution is accompanied by the risk of transmitting serum hepatitis.
  (d) Coagulation deficiencies in liver disease can be treated with fresh frozen plasma (FFP).
  (e) Factor VIII derived from freeze-dried concentrates has a half-life of 12 h in the circulation.

137 The following blood products are available:
  (a) Factor X concentrate.
  (b) Varicella zoster hyperimmune immunoglobulin.
  (c) Measles hyperimmune immunoglobulin.
  (d) Granulocyte concentrates.
  (e) Antithrombin III concentrate.

136 (a) **True**　The administration of albumin promotes a diuresis in diuretic-resistant nephrotic syndrome. This is the only definite indication because its value has not been proved in other hypoalbuminaemic states. It is presented as 100 ml of solution containing 20 g of albumin.

(b) **False**　They confer only passive immunity.

(c) **False**　Albumin solution is heated for 10 h at 60°C to inactivate the causative agent of serum hepatitis. It can be used in oligaemic shock and to replace protein loss following burns or crush injuries.

(d) **True**　FFP is valuable whenever there is depletion of several coagulation factors. It is used in liver disease, the treatment of haemorrhage due to coumarin drugs, haemorrhagic disease of the newborn and the dilutional coagulopathy following massive transfusion. It must be used as soon as it is thawed.

(e) **True**　Freeze-dried concentrates are the mainstay of the treatment for severe haemophilia A and have replaced cryoprecipitate. Virus inactivation by heat treatment or solvent detergent have minimised the risk of transmitting both HIV and hepatitis viruses. Immunoaffinity purified and recombinant DNA-derived factor VIII are now available but have not yet been shown to be superior to conventional intermediate purity factor VIII.

137 (a) **False**　Factor X-deficient patients are treated with factor IX concentrate, which currently also contains factors II and X.

(b) **True**　Zoster immune globulin (ZIG) is especially used to treat immunecompromised children exposed to chickenpox. Acyclovir has recently been used instead of ZIG in this setting.

(c) **False**　Although measles can be a life-threatening infection in immunocompromised children, this product is not available. Pooled immunoglobulin is given.

(d) **True**　The effectiveness of granulocyte transfusions in eradicating bacterial or fungal infections is not established. However, patients with severe neutropenia or abnormal neutrophil function with infection despite treatment with appropriate antibiotics for 72 h may be considered for a 3-day trial of granulocyte transfusions. If there is a good response the transfusions may be continued.

(e) **True**　Its main indication for use is the prevention of thrombosis in antithrombin III-deficient patients during surgery but its use in disseminated intravascular coagulation is under investigation.

138 Platelet concentrates:
   (a) Can be administered to ABO incompatible recipients.
   (b) Are ineffective if the patient has developed HLA antibodies.
   (c) Are non-contributory in treating bleeding where the platelet count is $> 100 \times 10^9/l$.
   (d) Are given prophylactically if the patient's platelet count is $< 20 \times 10^9/l$.
   (e) Should be stored at room temperature.

139 Plasmapheresis is therapeutically useful in the following situations:
   (a) Hyperviscosity syndrome associated with a paraprotein.
   (b) Cell-mediated immune disorders.
   (c) If a Rhesus (D) negative young woman is accidentally transfused with several units of Rhesus (D) positive blood.
   (d) To obtain platelets for therapeutic use.
   (e) In a young patient with homozygous sickle-cell disease who develops a stroke.

138 (a) **True** However ABO compatible, concentrates give greater platelet increments. Furthermore, ABO incompatible platelets may cause reactions due to red cell contamination or ABO agglutinins in the donor plasma. In addition, red cell contamination can stimulate Rhesus antibody formation and Rhesus-negative women of child-bearing age should receive Rhesus-negative platelet concentrates.

(b) **False** Random donor platelets may not cause an increment in the platelet count but HLA antibodies are weakly expressed on platelets, and in large quantities platelets may be useful. Prophylaxis with intravenous chlorpheniramine and hydrocortisone may prevent 'febrile transfusion reactions' in these patients. Ideally, HLA-matched platelets should be administered and leucodepleted blood products should be used as removal of white cells reduces febrile reactions and further alloimmunisation.

(c) **False** Some patients have dysfunctional platelets and benefit from random donor platelets. The functional defect may be congenital, e.g. Glanzmann's thromasthenia, or acquired, e.g. myeloproliferative, disorders.

(d) **True** This is common practice in patients with inadequate marrow-production of platelets, e.g. aplastic anaemia or receiving cytotoxic therapy.

(e) **True** Further improvement in platelet function and survival is achieved with storage in bags permitting gas transfer and if they are constantly agitated.

139 (a) **True** Care must be taken as the patients are often elderly and hypotension may be precipitated. Hyperviscosity is more likely with IgM or IgA paraproteins than IgG.

(b) **False** Removal of antibody by plasmapheresis is sometimes beneficial in antibody-mediated disorders, such as haemolytic disease of the newborn, myasthenia gravis and Goodpasture's syndrome.

(c) **False** Prompt red cell exchange and intramuscular anti-D in suitable quantities may avert sensitisation to the D antigen.

(d) **False** Many transfusion centres have a plateletpheresis donor clinic. These donors are able to donate more frequently than whole blood donors because red cells are not removed.

(e) **False** Red cell exchange with normal red cells is indicated in homozygous sickle-cell disease and in SC disease for a neurological event, chest/girdle syndrome and sometimes in pregnancy. Reduction of the circulating level of haemoglobin S to less than 30% of the total haemoglobin is required.

140 The following concern haemolytic disease of the newborn (HDN):
   (a) Rhesus haemolytic disease of the newborn is common in Rh(D) positive babies born to primiparous Rh(D) negative mothers.
   (b) Passively administered anti-D to Rh(D) negative mothers postpartum has reduced the incidence of Rh haemolytic disease.
   (c) High concentrations of unconjugated bilirubin can cause death.
   (d) A jaundiced neonate whose blood group is O and whose mother is group A could have haemolytic disease due to ABO incompatibility.
   (e) Exchange transfusion should always be performed in any newborn with haemolytic disease if the cord haemoglobin concentration is < 15 g/dl.

140 (a) **False**   Unless previously sensitised, anti-D can be detected in only 1% of Rh(D) negative mothers by the end of the first pregnancy. By the end of the second pregnancy with a Rh(D) positive infant, approximately 20% of Rh negative mothers will have developed detectable anti-D in their serum if they are not given prophylactic anti-D.

  (b) **True**   The routine intramuscular injection of 500 iu anti-D within 72 hours following delivery of the first child or 250 iu following early spontaneous abortion or termination of pregnancy, amniocentesis or external version, has reduced the incidence of anti-D antibodies developing to 1% or less at the end of the second pregnancy.

  (c) **True**   Unconjugated bilirubin is lipid-soluble and taken up by the brain. If the serum bilirubin concentration remains $> 300 \, \mu$mol/l in a full-term baby for longer than a few hours, kernicterus may develop. The outcome of this can be death, mental retardation, athetosis or deafness. In premature infants, kernicterus can occur at lower bilirubin concentrations.

  (d) **False**   A group O neonate's red cells do not contain A or B antigen. HDN due to ABO incompatibility is due to group A or B fetal cells crossing the placenta and stimulating the formation of increased amounts of maternal IgG anti-A or anti-B by group O mothers. The disease is usually mild and rarely, if ever, requires exchange transfusion.

  (e) **False**   Exchange transfusion is performed if the cord blood haemoglobin is < 11 g/dl or bilirubin $> 80 \, \mu$mol/l. After delivery a rise in serum bilirubin of $> 10 \, \mu$mol/l/h is an indication for exchange transfusion.

© 1992 T P Baglin, J E G Braithwaite, T R Mitchell

First published in Great Britain 1992

British Library Cataloguing in Publication Data

Baglin, T. P.
  Multiple choice questions in haematology.
  — 2nd ed.
  I. Title   II. Braithwaite, J. E. G.
  III. Mitchell, T. R.
  616.10076

  ISBN 0-340-55303-0

Whilst the advice and information in this book is believed to be true
and accurate at the date of going to press, neither the author nor the
publisher can accept any legal responsibility or liability for any errors
or omissions that may be made.

Typeset in Univers Light by Anneset, Weston-super-Mare, Avon.
Printed and bound in Great Britain for Edward Arnold, a division
of Hodder and Stoughton Limited, Mill Road, Dunton Green,
Sevenoaks, Kent TN13 2YA by Biddles Limited, Guildford and
King's Lynn.